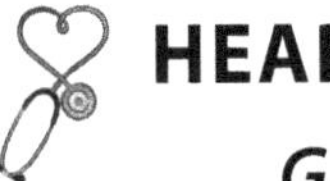

HEART SURGERY

Game Plan

HEART SURGERY
Game Plan

From Diagnosis Kickoff—
To Recovery Touchdown

YOUR PERSONAL STRATEGY FOR SUCCESS

Jacob DeLaRosa, M.D.

Heart Surgery Game Plan
From Diagnosis Kickoff—To Recovery Touchdown
Your Personal Strategy For Success

First Edition

Printed in the United States of America

Publishers Cataloging-in-Publication Data
DeLaRosa, Jacob
Heart Surgery Game Plan: From Diagnosis Kickoff to Recovery Touchdown, Your Personal Strategy for Success / Jacob DeLaRosa – 1st ed.
p. cm.
1. Health 2. Medicine

Softbound: ISBN-10: 1-880759-76-4 ISBN-13: 978-1-880759-76-9
Hardcover: ISBN-10: 1-880759-80-2 ISBN-13: 978-1-880759-80-6
eBook: ISBN-10: 1-880759-81-0 ISBN-13: 978-1-880759-81-3

DEDICATION

In life, we are fortunate if we find one coach to push, to inspire, and to make us believe in ourselves. I have been most blessed to have many "coaches" in my life who have brought out the best in me and challenged me to do better.

If it were not for the encouraging and sometimes bellowing cries of Don Aslett, this book would not have been completed. From the first day I met Don and he heard me speak, he has been after me to write and finish this book. He is a remarkable person, friend, and the best custodian I know. When Don got tired of beating on me, he sent the big gun, Sandra Phillips, after me. Sandi has been an amazing editor, friend, and, with a million things going on, the most organized person that I have ever met. Without her guidance this book would not have made it.

To my staff, especially my assistant Staccy. Without her help and organization this book would just be pages on the floor of my office.

To my family, friends, and colleagues who came to Idaho to be a part of this adventure. Many thought we were crazy for believing we could provide world-class heart care in a small city in Idaho. Well, we showed them! I especially want to thank Juan Leon for giving me the best anesthesia a gas passer can give; Joe Brown for drinking the punch and coming out with me; Janice Koehler for her positive attitude every other day; Julio Vasquez for the

Bruce Lee in him; Travis Elquist for his mullet hair; the Higgs for pumping it up; Bucholtz for the lemon drop; Pat Rasmussen for staying out of the room; Fernando Grigera for always looking debonair and ready to help; Amanda for the wax; Paige, Peggy, Joel, Michelle, and Mama for the amazing care they all provided; Sandy for her Rum cake; Steve Mclung for taking everything apart and then rebuilding it; Brandon for his respect; and Jason for his legendary West Coast exploits.

To my children Jacob IV, Giovanni, and Donatella. When I started writing this book there were only two of them. They are the joy that keeps me pushing ahead.

To my mother and father who believe in me every day and that I can do no wrong.

To all the patients that have allowed me the privilege to care for them, and who have put their lives in my hands.

Finally, to Mister. Without her daily support, friendship, and belief that I am her hero, these stories would not have happened. Off to the next adventure!!

—Jacob DeLaRosa, M.D.

TABLE OF CONTENTS

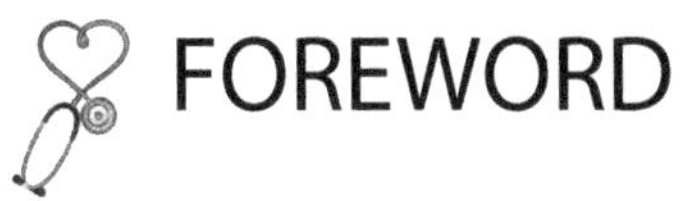

FOREWORD

Dinner With DeLaRosa

It was one of those days when I had ninety projects going on and no unscheduled time to complete them, but when my operations manager peeked her head in the door and asked, "Did you know Dr. DeLaRosa is speaking at the chamber dinner tonight at the Red Lion?" I decided to reallocate a few hours of my evening.

"That is no dinner, that is an *event*," I responded, picking up a yellow pad and flying out of the office—I was determined to be the first guest to arrive. The *event* was witnessing the impact of a world-class surgeon putting an insignificant Southern Idaho town on the map. Apparently, others shared my fascination for this doctor because the place filled from the usual fifty or sixty guests to more than 250.

Dr. DeLaRosa was introduced and the chattering crowd fell silent—intent to discover if he was as proficient with gab as he was at getting a heart healthy. As the young surgeon took the platform, a man at my table questioned why Dr. DeLaRosa was so willing to volunteer his time to speak. One of his associates responded, "That man is a giver, he doesn't need a whip, he needs a leash."

There are speakers and presenters, and then there are teachers and leaders. Dr. DeLaRosa left no doubt he was in the latter category. The combination of his confidence, his charisma, and the content of his presentation masterfully drove home the need to place better health as the world's number one priority. Heads were nodding in waves. The question and answer portion of his talk revealed warm humor and the unique character of this man. The collective groan from the audience following his revelation that he would telephone patients the day before surgery and give them his personal phone number came not from surprised guests but rather from the patients and friends at the dinner who already had his phone number!

When he finished speaking, emotional guests stood and thanked him for saving the lives of their sons or wives or friends. One young lady said, "Dr. DeLaRosa, because of you, my elderly mother is running on the beach in Miami." Dr. DeLaRosa quipped, "In her bikini?" The young woman came back, "No Doc, if she did, she'd cause more heart attacks."

Another voice piped up, "Trouble with you giving my wife a new life is now she loves you more than she loves me." Another person jumped to their feet, adding, "The great thing you've done, Dr. DeLaRosa, you brought a team—your team—as good as you are. Thank you!" I noticed ex-county commissioners in attendance who once voted against Dr. DeLaRosa's plans, but who were now his biggest supporters.

It is said that the mark of a great person is to have an instinct, a drive, a cause to bless mankind globally (not just his friends and family, or for money), and he will be active and generous in his "sphere of influences." The good Doctor wears those two badges well. That was a dinner of great, heartfelt digestion for all there and for the rest of the community Dr. DeLaRosa influences, which now reaches far beyond the little town of Pocatello.

—Don Aslett
Author, Inventor, Philanthropist
August 2011

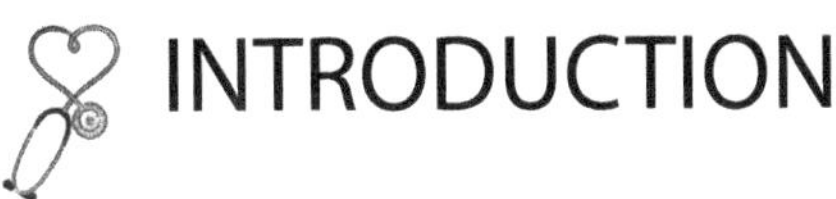

INTRODUCTION

The Kickoff

Growing up in Los Angeles, among the homes of celebrities and filmmakers, I was surrounded by the lure of glamour, the Hollywood lifestyle, and friends aspiring to attain the heights of stardom. But the glamorous life never held sway for me.

Starting from the age of five, my mother kept a diary of my exploits and adventures. She noted my first career choice was baseball player. A year later it had shifted to fireman. By the third grade, at the mature age of seven, I was determined to be a doctor. And that desire never wavered. Watching my physician father made me appreciate what it meant to be a healer and a helper.

I attended the University of Minnesota Medical School and did my general surgery residency at the University of California San Diego before moving on to Emory University for my residency in cardiothoracic (heart and lung) surgery. I noticed early on in my training that I didn't quite fit the mold of a physician, and especially not that of a surgeon. While many of my medical peers seemed aloof from patients, I made an effort to form a bond with them—I was quick with a joke and even quicker with a hug when needed.

It became apparent to me that as a health provider, I ought to listen to and understand patients, to take the time and responsibility to look after their spirits, and not just fix their hearts. I wanted to bring humanism into the mythical fascination of medicine. My attitude was controversial and my practices made me unpopular with other doctors and attending surgeons. I questioned whether I had made the right career choice. Then, in my second year of training in general surgery, I experienced a life-altering event.

I was preparing for an important exam and went for a quick jog to clear my head. As usual, I ran along the sidewalk of a residential area in La Jolla. I had my Walkman™ on and the volume turned up; I didn't hear the out-of-control vehicle approaching. As I sprinted into the cross walk, I was struck by a small truck traveling 60 miles-per-hour.

My body was tossed 100 feet from the impact site. I was unconscious when paramedics arrived and inserted a breathing tube. I was rushed to the hospital, where a chest tube was inserted. I had a collapsed lung, broken ribs, brain bleed, a shattered pelvis, and a broken right shoulder. I was non responsive.

Neurosurgeons evaluated the bleed in my brain and determined the bleeding was not expanding. I awoke several hours later to find my parents at my bedside. I had no recollection of the accident, and they had to explain what had happened. My lower extremities and right arm were in traction, and I had tubes coming out of my chest. I remember I was in dire need of water but was denied any fluids, as I was still considered critical.

Due to the extent of the trauma, I was transferred to the University Hospital under the care of Dr. David Hoyt where I was immediately taken to the operating room to fixate my pelvis and to repair my right shoulder. I awoke in the Intensive Care Unit with a breathing tube inside me. Breathing when one has a breathing tube in place is truly like breathing through a straw. It is very difficult to inhale. I understood why the tube was in place but that did not make it easier.

To say I was in pain is truly an understatement. When a bone is broken, every movement or motion causes extreme pain. While in the ICU it was hard to move as I lay on a plastic bed, pelvis fixated, right arm fixed, chest tube in my left chest, a catheter in place, and the worst headache imaginable. One day, while having my bed changed by a nurse, my catheter was ripped out of my penis. I screamed out in severe pain. The nurse's reaction? She told me to "shut up," as she did not understand what had happened.

I remained in the ICU for close to three weeks and was then transferred to another floor to continue healing. I was still unable to walk or move my right arm. Shortly after the transfer an incident occurred which was psychologically devastating, but at the same time it challenged me to take responsibility and act.

The attending physician and chief resident surgeon came to check on me, along with the trauma service, which consisted of more than seven doctors, two pharmacists, three medical students, one social worker, and one case manager. After the attending and chief resident concluded their examination and questions, they gathered in the corridor with the others on the team and I heard someone ask, "How is he?" The doctor replied, "He's fucked. He will never make it back."

I use my response to this situation in the way I practice medicine today. When I initially heard the doctor's prognosis, the wind was sucked out of me. I felt like Tom Cruise in the film, *Born on the Fourth of July*, when he is in rehab after being shot—sorry for myself, vulnerable, powerless, and depressed. I asked God why he had put me in this situation. I finally came to the realization nobody was going to get me going again except myself. I knew I had to start my own healing. I used the negative comments to fuel the fire inside of me. I was determined to prove them wrong.

I found a cheerleader in a physical therapist named Chris, a petite woman with a huge heart. She was the first to get me out of bed and make me stand on my legs. Still using my wheelchair, I began going outside and enjoying the sunlight. It was amazing for me to sit outside in the sun and absorb that energy. And even though I suffered many additional complications and another emergency surgery, I was able to leave the hospital six weeks after my initial accident and transfer to an inpatient rehabilitation center in San Diego.

Three moments stand out during my stay in rehabilitation: the first time I could walk (I felt liberated), when I had my first erection (I was told that I might never be able to have one again due to the trauma of the Foley catheter and the shattering of the pelvis), and when I took my first shower (until then I had only had sponge baths; today, I insist my patients be allowed to shower as soon as the second post-operative day).

Once I was finally released from rehabilitation and the metal cast from my pelvic fracture was removed, my parents took me to my home in San Diego. I insisted they return to their own home in Los Angeles, since they had already stayed with me for several months. I owe a tremendous gratitude to Dave and Pat Augustine who gave their home to my parents in San Diego during my lengthy hospitalization and recovery.

The next few days were the worst of my life. After that long hospitalization and being tended to constantly by nurses and staff, being home alone was extremely difficult. The depression was severe. After being home a week, I contacted my residency program director and told him I was ready to return to work. He advised me to take a year or two off to fully recover. I was adamant about returning. He agreed to evaluate me and, after doing so, cleared me to return to duty. I did not take any in-house calls that first month, but I was back—even after so many believed that I would not be.

Why was I able to recover when so many people in similar situations, and even people who suffered less severe trauma, could not? I analyzed my experience—as a surgeon, a patient, and now, as a survivor. I realized much of my success was due to my own determination and occurred in spite of the practices of many of my healthcare providers.

The lessons I learned from this experience form the basis for my medical practice today. All of my advice and patient coaching techniques flow from these five principles:

1. A patient's pain must be respected.
2. A patient's needs and requests should be examined on an individual basis and not simply dismissed due to an out-dated policy.
3. Listening to a patient and maintaining an open mind is imperative to ensure no diagnosis is over-looked.
4. Maintaining a positive attitude is essential for a patient's recovery. What is said and discussed by the staff taking care of a patient is critical.
5. Patients who are hospitalized long-term require the most care and attention once they leave the hospital. The highest rate of depression does not occur immediately after a trauma, or surgery, or even during the hospitalization. The highest rate of depression occurs upon going home.

Recovery from my accident was one of the most difficult times of my life but at the same time has made me the doctor I am today, the healer and the healthcare provider I strive to be. I know what it is like to be lying in bed, crippled, not able to go to the bathroom, peeing in a catheter, wearing gowns that open in the back, and listening to friends and colleagues question if you will ever "come back." I know what it takes to recover. I have been there and I made it!

I am reminded of my freshman basketball high school coach, Mike Graceffo, who said, "Never say, 'I can't'. Only losers say, 'I can't.' Winners say, 'I will try.'" When I found myself saying, "I can't…I can't walk, I can't use my arm, I can't bear the pain, I can't deal with the loneliness," I would stop myself, think of my coach, and say, "I will try." And I did, and I succeeded.

Any recovery is as much a patient's responsibility as the doctor's. As a physician I believe it is my role to push and to motivate, to be the cheerleader and the coach. Good coaches inspire, make you dream, make you believe in yourself, and give you the strength to accomplish anything.

This book is designed to give you that wakeup call before, not after the "problem." In it I will walk you through every step of your heart surgery process, from the initial diagnosis, to surgery, through recovery. Alongside your personal physician, I will be your personal coach, guiding you along the path, providing training, cheering you on, relaying advice, giving you pointers to create the best strategy for you, and sharing true tales (collected from my patient files) of strength, courage, and how to win the game when the odds seem against you.

This book is for you—the heart surgery player and survivor. Remember folks, you are *in* the "game"—not watching as a spectator !

Huddle up.

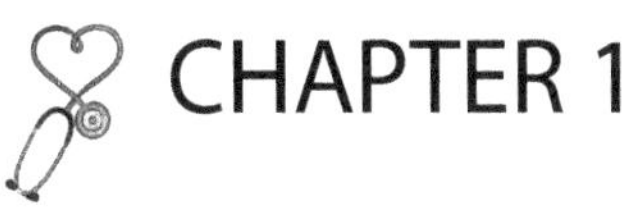

CHAPTER 1

Scouting The Opponent

Understanding Heart Disease

In any game, one of the most important elements is an understanding of the opponent. You can have the best training and skill in the world, but if you walk into a game without knowing exactly who and what you're up against, you're going to find yourself at a distinct disadvantage. Pure skill will not get you through the toughest competitions. You need to be able to anticipate your opponent's next move—to understand their inclinations and natural tendencies so you can always stay one step ahead.

To spot the weaknesses in your opponents you must scout and study them thoroughly. Scouting another team in order to find the holes in their defense or spot the open passing lanes against them has won many a football game for teams from high school to the NFL.

In many ways, the process of battling heart disease can take a form similar to that of preparing for the big game—probably the biggest game of your life. You may have a hard fight ahead of you but that in no way means you can't emerge victorious.

What you need to win this battle is knowledge. Just like a football scout, you need to study your opponent so that you know what you're facing and can devise a solid *game plan*. To take on heart disease, you need to first know how your heart works. You also need to understand the different types of heart disease and the various options for combating each of them.

Know this—heart disease is a fight you're capable of winning, and the first step is knowledge. As your coach, I'm going to guide you through scouting your opponent. It's not always fun, and it can be tedious, but having this awareness going into the game will make the victory that much easier.

HOW THE HEART WORKS

The basic function of the heart is to supply oxygen to the body. Your heart acts as a pump. The right side pumps blood to the lungs to pick up oxygen, the left side receives oxygen rich blood from the lungs and pumps it into the rest of the body.

A muscular organ about the size of your fist, the heart consists of four chambers, valves, and walls that separate the chambers. With

NORMAL HEART

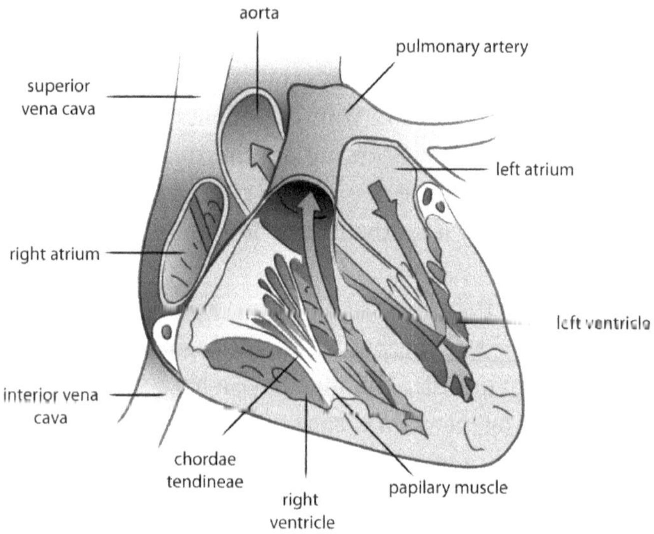

each beat, the heart receives, circulates, and delivers blood from the body and lungs. It has multiple branches that bring oxygenated and de-oxygenated blood to and from the heart and then distribute this blood to other organs.

Located in the chest cavity, the heart uses a nerve signal to create contractions. Coronary arteries wrap around the heart, supplying a continuous blood flow used by the heart for its own needs. In order for the heart to function properly, these coronary arteries must remain clear for blood flow. The heart beats 60 to 90 times per minute, and contracts about 100,000 times each day. It's always in the game—never resting or skipping practice.

THE HEART'S OXYGEN SUPPLY

As mentioned, the heart supplies its own nutrition. Even though the heart is full of blood, it receives its own oxygen-containing blood from arteries that extend from the aorta. Two coronary artery trunks stem from the root of the aorta. One of these is the right coronary artery, which supplies blood to the right ventricle and to several other sections of the left ventricle. The left main coronary artery divides into two more major coronary artery branches. The left anterior descending coronary artery provides blood to the front and the side of the left ventricle, as well as a wall of muscle tissue that divides the two ventricles.

When you're resting, the heart only has to pump enough oxygen-containing blood to the body to support your resting muscles and other organs. The oxygen requirement of the muscles of the body increases with exercise. Exercise causes your blood to move faster throughout your system, increases the force of each of your heartbeats, and decreases the resistance to blood flow in the arteries.

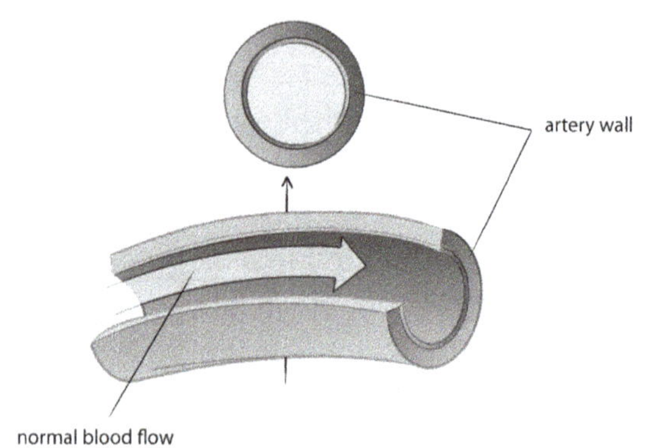

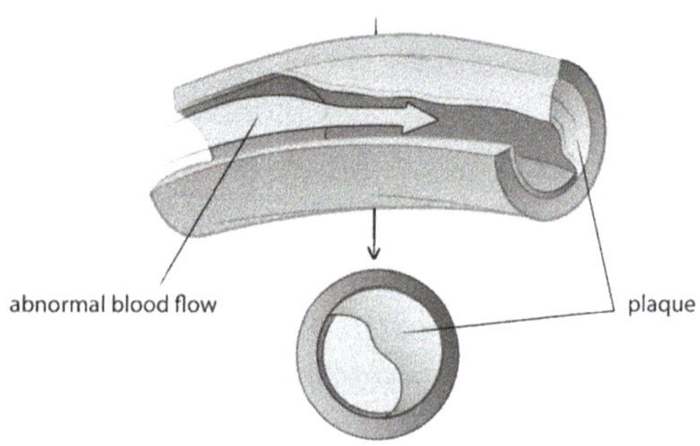

WHAT IS HEART DISEASE?

Heart disease is also known as cardiovascular disease or coronary artery disease, since it encompasses the heart, lungs, and vascular system. The vascular, or circulatory, system includes the arteries, veins, capillaries, and peripheral vessels that carry blood, nutrients, and fluid to every part of the body.

Coronary artery disease is caused when the coronary arteries become narrowed, and the heart muscle does not receive enough oxygen. Coronary artery disease causes angina (chest pain) and heart attacks. Over time, fatty materials, cholesterol, calcium, and other substances build up within the coronary arteries inner lining causing them to become blocked. This blockage is known as plaque.

Arterial plaque becomes distributed along the walls of arteries. It can accumulate more in some areas and less in others. You might have an 80% blockage in one small section of an artery.

For most people, arterial plaque builds over many years. Some build up has more cholesterol particles of plaque, while others have more hardened elements of plaque called fibrous tissue. Over time some plaque deposits may solidify or harden and reduce the flexibility the arteries need to help move blood throughout your body.

When the coronary arteries are healthy, exercise causes them to open so more blood gets to the heart muscle. But when coronary arteries are blocked, the blood supply to the heart is limited and, during exercise or moments of stress, the arteries are unable to dilate—leading to angina, unstable angina, and heart attacks.

A plaque rupture in one of the coronary arteries that supplies blood to the muscle of the heart is usually the initial event in a heart attack, which then leads to a localized clot that completely blocks the blood flow to part of the heart muscle.

ATHEROSCLEROSIS

Coronary artery disease is a precursor to developing atherosclerosis. Atherosclerosis is a hardening of the arterial or vascular walls. This hardening leads to increases in blood pressure, resting heart rate, and an enlarging of the heart due to increased workload. Over time, plaque hardens and narrows the arteries, reducing the flow of oxygen-rich blood to the organs and other parts of the body. This can lead to serious heart problems, including heart attack or stroke.

HOW HEART DISEASE AFFECTS OTHER AREAS OF THE BODY

Arteries bring oxygen-rich blood to every major organ in your body, not just the heart.

- **The brain:** Blockages in the carotid and vertebral arteries cause reduced blood flow to the brain. This critical lack of oxygen can cause a stroke in which some brain cells die.
- **The kidneys:** Very few people relate kidneys to heart health; however, when the renal arteries, which feed your kidneys, become partially blocked, the kidneys raise your blood pressure.
- **The legs:** When the muscles and tissues of your legs do not receive enough blood, you may experience cramping or muscle weakness during exercise. Over time the pain may become more constant and is an indication you are at greater risk for a heart attack or stroke.

SYMPTOMS OF CORONARY ARTERY DISEASE

Angina

The first sign of coronary artery disease is often angina. As mentioned before, angina is a chest pain that occurs during exercise, exertion, or emotional stress. Angina is experienced as a dull, heavy, constricting sensation that starts in the center of the chest and may spread into the throat or down one arm. In women, the symptoms are usually different, with feelings of nausea, shortness of breath and the sensation of heartburn. Angina usually disappears within 10 minutes of rest. When you stop exercising and rest your heart, it requires less oxygen to support the reduced level of activity. However, if your body cannot correct the imbalance then some of the cells in the heart that have been starved of oxygen will become injured and some may actually die; this death leads to a heart attack.

If the blockage in the coronary arteries is severe, angina may be experienced even when resting. If your angina reaches this level it becomes a serious condition called unstable angina. Patients who develop severe angina are likely to experience a heart attack within a few weeks or a few months. There is also a form of painless angina, sometimes experienced as being out-of-breath, which is only detected by an electrocardiogram (ECG).

Cardiac Arrest

Cardiac arrest is a sudden, complete loss of heart function. Death may occur within 4 to 6 minutes after someone goes into cardiac arrest. An irregular heart rhythm causes the heart to suddenly stop beating. A patient can be brought out of cardiac arrest if treated within the first few minutes with an electrical shock or defibrillation to the heart, which helps restore the normal heartbeat.

Heart Attack

Most heart attacks happen in the following sequence:

1. Pain occurs in the central part of the chest or in the neck or back, along with one arm, or in the elbows. Sometimes you may feel pain in your teeth or jaw. In women it can be a feeling of extreme nausea.
2. Shortness of breath may be acute.
3. Your body's sympathetic nervous system is activated, releasing chemicals, including adrenaline, that prepare your body for trauma. This makes the heart pump faster and harder, and your heart now requires even more oxygen. This stresses your heart's cells even further, and the demand for oxygen continues to increase.
4. Blood pressure rises. The major arteries constrict in order to move blood out of less critical areas and into more criti-

cal areas, such as the muscles and brain. This causes your blood pressure to rise and make the plaque in the coronary arteries more likely to rupture.

When a heart attack occurs, the coronary artery is blocked suddenly and completely, causing an area of muscle to die. Many heart attacks occur in patients with no previous warning signs of angina. And up to 25% of heart attacks have no corresponding chest pain. These *silent heart attacks* are common in patients with diabetes.

Symptoms that may indicate heart attack

- Severe heavy crushing pain in the chest
- A pain in the chest that may feel like a squeezing pressure
- Pain that does not go away with rest
- Difficulty breathing
- Rapid heartbeat
- Pain that lasts more than 20 to 30 minutes
- Cramps in the legs during exercise may indicate arterial plaque is decreasing blood supply to the major muscles of your legs
- Chest pain, associated with exercise or stress
- Shortness of breath
- Discomfort in the upper body—including one or both arms, the back, neck, jaw, or stomach
- A cold sweat
- A hot or flushed feeling
- Racing or fluttering heart
- Nausea (women)

Symptoms of a stroke

- Sudden numbness or weakness in the face, arm, or leg, especially on one side of the body
- Confusion or trouble speaking
- A sudden visual change in one or both eyes
- Dizziness, difficulty walking, loss of balance or coordination
- A sudden, severe headache
- Loss of consciousness

Many people do not notice any symptoms until they experience their first cardiovascular event, such as a heart attack or a stroke.

In the event of a heart attack, getting to the hospital quickly is crucial. Doctors can take immediate steps to prevent further blood clots, decrease your heart rate and blood pressure to reduce the excess demand of the heart for oxygen, and ideally remove a blockage to restore some blood flow.

What Happens to the Heart After a Heart Attack?

After experiencing a heart attack:

- Scar tissue is formed. Damaged heart muscle cells are replaced with scar tissue during the healing process. This scar tissue does not contract to pump blood.
- Heart muscle thickens. The tissue surrounding the scar tissue compensates for the lost pumping power. Because it is working harder, it becomes thicker and stronger.
- The ventricles will dilate. If the ventricle is unable to pump out enough blood to feed the body's organs and tissues, the muscle tissue will stretch and dilate under the pressure of the blood entering the ventricle. This condition leads to heart failure.

Heart Failure

Heart failure can occur when the heart can no longer pump adequate amounts of blood. A normal ventricle pumps out 50% to 70% of its blood with every contraction. When contraction is reduced to less than 40% or 30%, symptoms of heart failure occur. The heart becomes larger. Its reduced ability to pump blood causes blood to pool in the lungs and extremities and leads to swelling of the legs or generalized bloating in the body, along with fatigue and shortness of breath.

OTHER HEART CONDITIONS

Heart Valve Degeneration

Each year about five million Americans will learn they have heart valve disease. There are several causes of heart valve degeneration; these include bacterial infection, birth defects, rheumatic fever, and the natural aging process. There are four valves in your heart that control the flow of blood between the chambers of the heart and between the heart and the rest of the body. When the heart is functioning properly these valves open to allow blood to pass through into the next chamber and then close off completely to keep any of that blood from flowing back.

Stenosis of a heart valve occurs when the valve is unable to open all the way, and the blood must be forced through a narrower opening than normal. This means the heart muscles will have to pump harder or more frequently to move the blood through the damaged valve. I like to think of it as watering the grass while your thumb is over the end of the hose and the water is being held back with increased pressure. This puts added strain on the heart and can lead to other problems. Also, if the heart is not strong enough to compensate for the smaller opening, blood flow throughout the body may become insufficient.

Regurgitation, on the other hand, is a problem that occurs when a valve has degenerated to the point where it is unable to close fully. This allows some blood to pass back through the opening, resulting in a smaller volume of blood being moved along with each contraction of the heart muscle. This condition will also cause your heart to have to work harder to move the same amount of blood as it did before, leading to the same types of complications as stenosis.

For many, there are no exhibiting symptoms of heart valve disease, but others may experience chest pain, foot swelling, dizziness, shortness of breath, fainting, and fatigue. Valves function like the snap of the ball for a quarterback. If timing isn't flawless, it can cause a false start, offsides, or a failed scramble.

Congenital Heart Defects

A congenital heart defect is an abnormality in the formation or functioning of the heart that is present from birth. It is estimated that nearly 1.3 million Americans may suffer from this anomaly. There are many types of congenital heart defects, and they vary a great deal in terms of severity. Some congenital heart defects can go unnoticed for many years because they do not interfere with the normal functioning of the body and produce no symptoms. Other defects are immediately life-threatening from the moment of birth.

Hypoplasia

One of the most serious types of congenital heart defect is called hypoplasia. Babies born with this condition have only one adequately developed ventricle and so are unable to move blood either throughout the body (left ventricle) or into the lungs (right ventricle). This condition is immediately life-threatening and requires emergency surgery. Generally this type of defect is discovered at birth or very soon after and must be treated immediately.

Obstruction Defects

Some other congenital heart defects fall under the category of obstruction defects. These can take many forms and affect different areas in the heart. Generally, an obstruction defect involves an unnatural narrowing of the valves or coronary arteries. These types of defects can be minor or life-threatening depending on the extent to which they restrict blood flow. Many minor obstruction defects go unnoticed for many years by the people who have them.

Septal Defects

Another type of congenital heart defect is a septal defect. People with septal defects have an abnormality in the septum, or the dividing wall between the right and left sides of the heart. These types of defects generally take the form of a hole that can allow blood to pass from the right to the left side and lessen the efficiency of the heart, but they also cover a wide range in terms of severity. Like obstruction defects, septal defects can be immediately life-threatening or produce no noticeable symptoms at all.

Arrhythmia

Also known as cardiac dysrhythmia, an arrhythmia is a disruption in the normal rhythm of the heart caused by irregular electrical activity. Some types of arrhythmias are life-threatening, while others may be frightening but pose no actual threat to life. Only your doctor will be able to tell if your arrhythmia is a sign of a potentially life-threatening underlying condition.

One example of an arrhythmia is bradycardia—a condition characterized by a heart rate of less than 60 beats a minute in an adult. This is not often an immediately life-threatening type of arrhythmia, but it can lead to other problems if it is allowed to persist. This type of arrhythmia is often treated with the implantation of a pacemaker to regulate the heart's electrical activity.

The opposite of bradycardia, tachycardia, is defined as a heart rate of over 100 beats per minute in an adult. There are many reasons for tachycardia, and not all of them are life-threatening, but persistent tachycardia can begin to cause other serious problems throughout the body and should be investigated and treated by a doctor.

Fibrillation is a more serious and life-threatening form or arrhythmia and requires immediate medical attention. Fibrillation can affect either the atrium or the ventricle on either side of the heart and will result in the heart not being able to pump blood effectively to the lungs or the rest of the body.

In order to determine the exact nature and extent of an arrhythmia, your doctor will have to perform an electrocardiogram, a test that can be used to evaluate the electrical activity in the heart. Depending on the type and severity of your arrhythmia, the type of treatment that is appropriate can vary a great deal.

RISK FACTORS

Risk factors are categorized as controllable or non-controllable. Controllable risk factors include smoking, obesity, and inactivity. Non-controllable factors include age, gender, and family history.

Genetics & Heredity

If your parents or other family members have heart disease then you are at higher risk for developing the condition.

Age & Gender

The risk of experiencing a heart attack increases with age. Men are at greater risk after the age of 45. For women, their risk increases after menopause. Heart disease is the leading cause of death for both men and women.

According to the American Heart Association, one in eight women aged 45 to 64 has heart disease. One in four women over the age of 65 has heart disease. Currently 7.2 million women have heart disease.

According to the Mayo Clinic, men suffer from heart disease 10 to 15 years earlier than women, and they're more likely to die of it in the prime of life. About 25% of all heart disease related deaths occur in men between the ages of 35 and 65.

Smoking

Smoking is the most dangerous risk factor. Smokers are 3 to 5 times more likely to die of heart disease than non-smokers. Lungs soak up the tar and carcinogenic particles, which are then deposited into the soft tissues. The lungs are responsible for converting deoxygenated blood for use throughout the body via the heart's pumping mechanism. Once the lungs are polluted with chemicals, the capacity to oxygenate blood is greatly decreased, leading to the development of diseases such as chronic obstructive pulmonary disease (COPD), bronchitis, emphysema, and congestive heart failure. A first heart attack is more likely to be fatal if you smoke. The first training rule for any great athlete is to ditch the cigarettes—and it should be your first training rule, too.

Cholesterol

Cholesterol is a naturally occurring substance that circulates throughout all parts of the body. Cholesterol has many functions, including the production of cell membranes, hormonal regulation, and the functioning of the nervous system. Certain foods can cause excessive cholesterol buildup in the arterial walls leading to hypertension, coronary artery disease, heart attack, and stroke. Because cholesterol and other fatty substances cannot be dissolved in the bloodstream, they are transported to cells by lipoprotein.

Low-density lipoprotein (LDL) is referred to as bad cholesterol, and high-density lipoprotein (HDL) is known as good cholesterol. A high level of LDL particles, or bad cholesterol, leads to the progression of heart disease. HDL, or good cholesterol, protects against heart disease; a low level increases risk. A healthy or normal range for cholesterol is less than 100 mg of LDL and more than 50 mg of HDL.

Sedentary Lifestyle

Exercise is essential for protecting your cardiovascular system from disease. It burns sugar and fat, which reduces your risk of arterial plaque. It also improves circulation and increases the oxygen in your blood.

Obesity / BMI

According to a study published in the *New England Journal of Medicine*, having a large waistline can almost *double* your risk of dying prematurely, even if your body mass index is within the normal range. Increases in waist circumference can indicate a greater amount of belly fat, which has been linked to the development of metabolic syndrome and cardiovascular disease.

BODY MASS INDEX

WEIGHT	lbs	100	105	110	115	120	125	130	135	140	145	150	155	160	165	170	175	180	185	190	195	200	205	210	215
	kgs	45.5	47.7	50.0	52.3	54.5	56.8	59.1	61.4	63.6	65.9	68.2	70.5	72.7	75.0	77.3	79.5	81.8	84.1	86.4	88.9	90.9	93.2	95.5	97.7
HEIGHT in/cm			Underweight					Healthy					Overweight					Obese				Extremely obese			
5'0"	152.4	19	20	21	22	23	24	25	26	27	28	29	30	31	32	33	34	35	36	37	38	39	40	41	42
5'1"	154.9	18	19	20	21	22	23	24	25	26	27	28	29	30	31	32	33	34	35	36	36	37	38	39	40
5'2"	157.4	18	19	20	21	22	22	23	24	25	26	27	28	29	30	31	32	33	33	34	35	36	37	38	39
5'3"	160.0	17	18	19	20	21	22	23	24	24	25	26	27	28	29	30	31	32	32	33	34	35	36	37	38
5'4"	162.5	17	18	18	19	20	21	22	23	24	24	25	26	27	28	29	30	31	31	32	33	34	35	36	37
5'5"	165.1	16	17	18	19	20	20	21	22	23	24	25	25	26	27	28	29	30	30	31	32	33	34	35	35
5'6"	167.6	16	17	17	18	19	20	21	21	22	23	24	25	25	26	27	28	29	29	30	31	32	33	34	34
5'7"	170.1	15	16	17	18	10	19	20	21	22	22	23	24	25	25	26	27	28	29	29	30	31	32	33	33
5'0"	172.7	15	16	16	17	18	19	19	20	21	22	22	23	24	25	25	26	27	28	28	29	30	31	32	32
5'9"	175.2	14	15	16	17	17	18	19	20	20	21	22	22	23	24	25	25	26	27	28	28	29	30	31	31
5'10"	177.8	14	15	15	16	17	18	18	19	20	20	21	22	23	23	24	25	25	26	27	28	28	29	30	30
5'11"	180.3	14	14	15	16	16	17	18	18	19	20	21	21	22	23	23	24	25	25	26	27	28	28	29	30
6'0"	182.8	13	14	14	15	16	17	17	18	19	19	20	21	21	22	23	23	24	25	25	26	27	27	28	29
6'1"	185.4	13	13	14	15	15	16	17	17	18	19	19	20	21	21	22	23	23	24	25	25	26	27	27	28
6'2"	187.9	12	13	14	14	15	16	16	17	18	18	19	19	20	21	21	22	23	23	24	25	25	26	27	27
6'3"	190.5	12	13	13	14	15	15	16	16	17	18	18	19	20	20	21	21	22	23	23	24	25	25	26	26
6'4"	193.0	12	12	13	14	14	15	15	16	17	17	18	18	19	20	20	21	22	22	23	23	24	25	25	26

Diabetes

Patients with diabetes are at higher risk of developing cardiovascular disease. It is estimated that approximately 65% of diabetics die from cardiovascular disease.

Types of diabetes:

- **Type I Diabetes:** This results from the body's failure to produce insulin, the hormone that unlocks the cells of the body, allowing glucose to enter and fuel them. About 10% of Americans who are diagnosed with diabetes have type I diabetes.
- **Type II Diabetes:** This results from insulin resistance, a condition in which the body fails to properly use insulin, combined with relative insulin deficiency. The majority of Americans diagnosed with diabetes have type II diabetes.

Blood Sugar

High levels of blood sugar, or glucose, increase risk of heart disease. In a healthy body, sugar circulates for a short period of time through the bloodstream and then insulin converts it into fuel that your cells store and use later. For people who suffer from high blood sugar, glucose circulates for an extended period of time through the bloodstream damaging organs in the body. If you have type I diabetes you will need to monitor your insulin dosage to optimize glucose control. If you have type II diabetes you will need to strictly control your diet and ensure you get plenty of exercise.

Stress

For people who suffer from heart disease, daily stressful activities such as emotional confrontations, episodes of extreme anger, and stressful situations can lead to sudden heart attacks. Tension and anger rapidly increase your heart rate and blood pressure, thus increasing your heart's need for oxygen. If arteries are blocked, the heart will not receive enough oxygen. This lack of oxygen can lead to a heart attack.

Stress is a primary risk factor that can lead to hypertension, and ultimately a pro-inflammatory state where your body becomes increasingly susceptible to inflammation. Long-term inflammation can eventually weaken your circulatory system and decrease your body's immune system.

The Miller and Smith Stress Test

Directions: score each item from one (always) to five (never), according to how much of the time each statement applies to you.

1 *(always)* 4 *(almost never)*
2 *(almost always)* 5 *(never)*
3 *(periodically)*

1. ___ I eat at least one hot, balanced meal a day.
2. ___ I get 7 to 8 hours of sleep, at least four nights each week.
3. ___ I give and receive affection regularly.
4. ___ I have at least one relative within 50 miles.
5. ___ I exercise to the point of perspiration at least twice each week.
6. ___ I smoke less than half a pack of cigarettes a day.
7. ___ I drink fewer than five alcoholic drinks per week.
8. ___ I am the appropriate weight for my height.
9. ___ I have an income adequate to meet basic expenses.
10. ___ I receive strength from my religious beliefs.
11. ___ I regularly attend club or social activities.
12. ___ I have a network of friends and acquaintances.
13. ___ I have one or more friends to confide in about personal matters.
14. ___ I am in good health (including eyesight, hearing, and teeth).
15. ___ I am able to speak openly about my feelings when angry or worried.
16. ___ I have regular conversations with the people I live with about domestic problems, chores, money, and daily living issues.
17. ___ I do something for fun at least once a week.
18. ___ I am able to organize my day effectively.
19. ___ I drink fewer than 3 cups of coffee (or tea, or cola drinks) each day.
20. ___ I take quiet time for myself during the day.

TOTAL RAW SCORE: _____
TOTAL RAW SCORE – 20 = ____ (Vulnerability Score)

To calculate your score, add all of the numbers and subtract 20. Any number over 30 indicates a vulnerability to stress. You are seriously vulnerable if your score is between 50 and 75, and extremely vulnerable if it is over 75.

High Blood Pressure or Hypertension

High blood pressure can be caused by genetics, stress, or eating a diet high in fat. High blood pressure affects about 30% of Americans, and if left untreated, can damage arteries, which can lead to blood clots, strokes, and heart disease. When you have high blood pressure, your heart has to pump harder and the arteries are under increased pressure, which can lead to injury of the artery walls and coronary heart disease.

Blood pressure is the force of blood pushing against the blood vessel walls. The measurement consists of two numbers: the top number (systolic blood pressure) measures the pressure when the heart beats; the bottom number (diastolic blood pressure) measures the pressure when the heart rests between beats. A high blood pressure is considered to be 140 systolic or 90 diastolic.

A healthy blood pressure is considered to be 120/80. According to the Princeton Medical Center, for every 20 point increase in systolic and 10 point increase in diastolic blood pressure, your risk for developing coronary heart disease doubles.

A healthy heart should be the concern of doctor and patient alike. Until we treat the heart as the quarterback of the whole body, we cannot expect good health or a long life.

Evaluating Your Risk Factors

- What is my cholesterol level?
- What can I do to reduce my cholesterol level?
- What is my level of exercise?
- How can I add exercise to my daily routine?
- What is my blood sugar level?
- What is my blood pressure?
- Am I a smoker?
- If I smoke, am I committed to quitting?
- Am I at risk for developing heart failure?

- What symptoms should I be aware of?
- How much of a role does stress play in my life?
- How can I reduce the stress level in my life?

LET THE GAME BEGIN

A Personal Story Of Launching An Innovative Heart Program

In launching a new state-of-the-art heart surgery program, I spent many hours making sure everything was just right. In early winter 2004, I went out to Pocatello, in Southeast Idaho, to get the job started and carefully selected a team of support individuals. No detail was overlooked in preparing the heart program. I was set on making this heart program world-class. Unfortunately, the reasoning of, "If you build it, they will come," was not going to be why patients would come see us.

Society is sophisticated enough to realize that a center that is treating the sickest of patients has to have good results or people will not come. Most new programs close down in their first year if they don't approach the situation carefully and methodically. New programs shoot for the zero/one hundred rule. This means zero mortality in one hundred cases. This is an unwritten rule, but a standard for which new programs to strive. To reach this goal, patients are carefully selected and screened to have minimal risk factors for maximal outcomes. This "ultimate patient" can be elusive, and just the desire to get started can be overwhelming.

I enticed my Anesthesiologist, Dr. Joe Brown, and my O.R. Manager, Caryn Buckholtz, to come with me to Pocatello and help with this new adventure. I had realized early on in my career that no matter how talented or gifted the surgeon, the results depend on a good team.

Dr. Brown gave up a lucrative practice in Charleston, South Carolina, to join me. When I first called Joe one year earlier, I was in Atlanta driving my car to the hospital. I knew that Joe was the right man for the job, as I had worked with him at Emory. He was impressive, knowledgeable, and had what most anesthesiologists lack—a compassionate heart. He was the right man for the job.

As we spoke on the phone, I said, "Joe, I need you. I need help."

"Jake, do you need some money?" he asked.

"No, I need you!" I replied. I explained to him what I was planning to start in Idaho, and he was excited but had his reservations. Joe was a newlywed to a debutante from Atlanta. Her notion of roughing it was a Four Seasons Hotel without a spa. Nevertheless, Joe and his wife came out to Pocatello to visit and fell in love with the small town and rural atmosphere; besides, Nordstrom was only 170 miles away in Salt Lake City. Having Joe join me, I knew we would be unstoppable. I respected what he did, and he respected what I did.

Caryn was also a strategic member of the team. Like Joe, I knew Caryn from Emory and respected what she did. Again, most would say that her job as the manager of the operating room is small compared to what I do, but without her, I cannot do what I do. Every person is only as great as his or her support team. Caryn left Emory one year earlier when she went off to Harvard to do her craft. She did such an amazing job at the Brigham and Women's hospital that they begged her to stay.

Caryn was single, and I realized that Pocatello, Idaho, was not the most happening of places compared to Boston, Los Angeles, or Atlanta, but in order for us to succeed, I needed her attitude and her expertise. Caryn was young, but had "heart," and her inexperience would be overshadowed by her desire to make this program excel, which it did! Before Caryn arrived, the operating room was unfinished. By opening day, she had transformed a blank canvas into a masterpiece.

On every journey one needs a compadre to share in the adventure and the excitement. If one does it alone it is only half as fun. Having my infrastructure set and my anesthesiologist at the head, I next needed an exceptional assistant to be my trusted compadre. That slot was filled by someone whom many call the "City Girl," Jan Koehler. Jan was also from the Emory system and was one hell of a Physician's Assistant. She has compassion, knowledge, excellent decision-making capabilities, and superior judgment.

Jan was the head P.A. at Emory University under Dr. Joseph Craver. Dr. Craver was tall, fit, and afraid of nothing and no one. He ran the show at Emory, and he was also an outstanding surgeon. Dr. Craver was an excellent mentor who had many "Craverisms."

I remember once opening a re-do, re-do, re-do chest for a valve operation. (What that means is that the chest had been operated on three times prior.) This operation is dangerous and challenging. Every time the chest is opened, it heals with scar tissue. The normal surgical plane no longer exists, and the risks of sawing through the heart when opening the chest are high. This patient had between a 60% to 70% chance of dying or having a serious complication.

I opened the chest with meticulous care and safety. When Dr. Craver walked into the operating room I said to him, "That was a really hard chest I opened, but she is doing great." He looked at me as he towered over me by five inches, like a middle linebacker about to pounce on the offense. (By the way, did I mention that Dr. Craver was an All-American football player?) In his deep, rough voice he said, "Jake, self-praise is no praise." I never forgot that Craverism and often think before I speak about a triumph or an accomplishment.

Jan respected Dr. Craver, as he was truly an outstanding surgeon who had no fear and operated on the sickest of sick, but she also saw something in me. In the operating room, Jan and I work together in harmony like the Boston Symphony. Jan made major sacrifices to leave Atlanta and join me. Professionally, she was the chief P.A. at a world-class heart center that was top in the United States, and she was stepping down. Personally, her significant other did not want to leave Atlanta, so Jan apologized but said this was her calling to help in Pocatello, Idaho.

Three months passed since Jan had made the big move to the budding metropolis of Pocatello, and I returned to Atlanta for a visit. Dr. Craver called me into his office and asked me how everything was in Idaho, with my family, etc. He questioned why I took Jan without asking his permission. I tried to explain, but he would not let me get a word in, and you don't push a man who has dead animals hanging on his walls. He told me he was disappointed in me for not saying anything to him. I responded, finally getting a word in, "Dr. Craver, it was not an option." I knew he would have said no, and even if Jan did not want to stay he still would have said no.

Dr. Craver understood, and he was not upset because she was with me, but I felt he was upset because he had lost, finally! I truly love Dr. Craver for everything he taught me about life and heart surgery, and I know he is proud of what we have done. Jan is my assistant, but she is also my friend and colleague, and, to borrow the cliché, "She completes me" in the O.R.

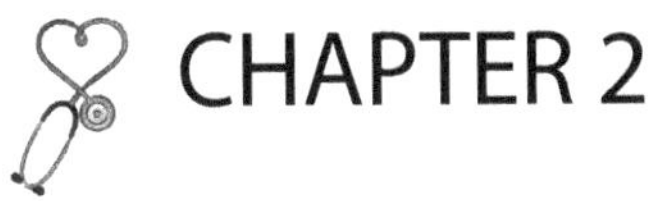

CHAPTER 2

The Game Plan

Understanding Your Diagnosis And Surgical Options

Once you have a basic understanding of how the heart works and the problems it can have, you're ready to start putting together a game plan with your doctors and others.

Tackling heart disease is necessarily a group effort. Your ability to emerge from this fight victorious will be a direct result of the coordinated efforts of you, your family and friends, your doctor, and the other medical professionals involved in your care.

The best way to make sure everyone is working together efficiently toward victory is to lay out a thorough game plan. Think of this as a series of plays, each of which will be set up to address a certain aspect of the opponent, your heart disease. Don't wait until the coin toss at the start of the game to start planning your plays—every player needs to be prepared before stepping onto the field.

Your opening drive will mostly be designed to feel out your opponent and get a sense of the dimensions of your disease. An evaluation of your symptoms and a battery of diagnostic tests will usually be in order at the beginning of this process. You will work particularly closely with your doctor and keep the lines of communication open at all times. That way, your doctor will be able to analyze exactly the severity of your disease.

Once you've gathered this information, you will be in a better position to challenge your opponent directly. You and the other members of your team will be able to decide which treatment avenue to pursue, and what an appropriate timeline for that treatment will be.

Getting into the lead by designing an effective treatment plan is only half the battle. You'll need to make sure the plan includes plays for holding onto that lead into the waning moments of the game. To come out a winner, you need to know what types of situations might develop later in the game and have a play ready to address each of them.

EXAMINING THE CONDITION OF YOUR HEART

Cardiologists are specialists in analyzing heart conditions but do not necessarily operate on the heart, although that is changing. If you are showing signs of heart disease or have determined you are at high risk for heart disease there is an assortment of tests and tools they will use to examine your heart condition.

If your physician thinks you have angina, there are a number of ways to confirm that you have it, find out the reason for it, and decide how serious it is. Your physician may prescribe lipid-lowering medication to slow down the progression of atherosclerosis throughout your body, aspirin to reduce the risk of having a heart attack by thinning the blood, and anti-angina drugs to relieve your angina symptoms. You may also undergo some of the following noninvasive tests that will show how your heart is working. Your doctor is your coach, and these tests will help him or her see what the *play* options are.

Cardiac Stress Test

This is a test of your heart function after a standardized amount of exertion.

Exercise Stress Echo

During this test, doctors monitor you and your heart while you exercise on a treadmill or stationary bicycle.

Nuclear Perfusion Scan

In this test, a radioactive isotope is injected into your body to measure the flow of blood. This test is used to diagnose angina. It can be done in addition to, or before, an angiogram, which is also known as angiography. This test is often used for people who are unable to exercise on a treadmill.

Echocardiogram

This is an ultrasound image of the inside of your heart. It is used to examine the size and function of heart structures and to diagnose heart disorders. A graphic outline is produced of the heart's movement, valves, and chambers using high-frequency sound waves delivered from a handheld wand placed on the outside of your chest. It is a painless process. An echocardiogram is often combined with Doppler ultrasound and color Doppler to evaluate blood flow across the heart valves.

Transesophageal Echocardiogram

This test is similar to an echocardiogram, but a 1-inch plastic tube is inserted into your mouth down your swallowing tube (esophagus) so excellent images of your heart are obtained.

Electrocardiogram (EKG or ECG)

This test records on graph paper the electrical activity of your heart via small electrode patches attached to the skin. An EKG helps the doctor determine the causes of an abnormal heartbeat or detect heart damage.

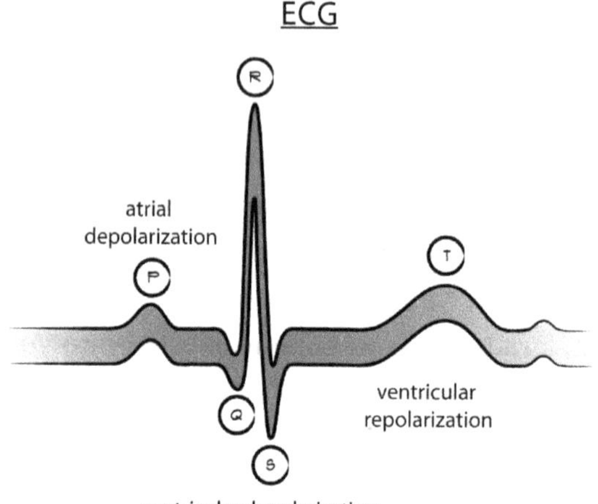

Angiography Or Cardiac Catheterization (Heart Cath)

A heart cath is an invasive imaging procedure that usually involves inserting a catheter into an artery leading to the heart muscle and injecting dye into the bloodstream. This test is used to determine if there is fatty buildup or plaque in the arteries that is causing narrowing. Cardiac catheterization is also referred to as a coronary angiography.

A heart cath gives a clear picture of your heart disease to your physician so he can recommend a treatment that is right for you.

Preparing for the procedure

- *Do not eat or drink for 6 hours prior to arriving at the hospital, except for medications as directed.*
- *Take a sip of water with all your medications.*
- *Blood-thinning medication must be stopped 3 to 5 days before your procedure (unless instructed otherwise by your physician).*
- *Be sure to inform your doctor if you are allergic to contrast dye or shellfish. If you have back problems, inform your doctor before you go into the cath lab.*

Your heart catheter procedure will be performed in the cath lab. When you arrive at the hospital and have changed into a hospital gown, a nurse will weigh you, check your vital signs, and insert an intravenous line into a vein in one of your arms. This will be used to give you fluids and to administer drugs during and after your procedure. Your physician will then examine you.

Your groin area will be shaved, and routine blood tests will be performed to check that your kidneys are working and that you are not anemic. An ECG will also be performed. (You may have already gone through a few of these steps during previous hospital visits.) If you have any final unanswered questions, be sure to ask the nurse who is assigned to you.

Questions to ask about your heart catheter procedure

- *Why do I need a heart cath?*
- *What will happen if blockages are found in my arteries?*
- *If I need an angioplasty, will it be done right away or will I need to come back?*
- *What are the risks?*
- *How long does the procedure take?*
- *Will I be awake for the procedure?*
- *How long will I need to stay in the hospital afterward?*
- *When will I be able to return to work?*

When you reach the cardiac catheterization laboratory, you will be introduced to all the staff in addition to your main physician. There will be nurses and technicians to answer any questions. The lab temperature is usually cool to ensure reliable running of the x-ray and recording equipment. You will be positioned on a narrow x-ray table and covered in sterile drapes. If you need addi-

CARDIAC CATHETERIZATION

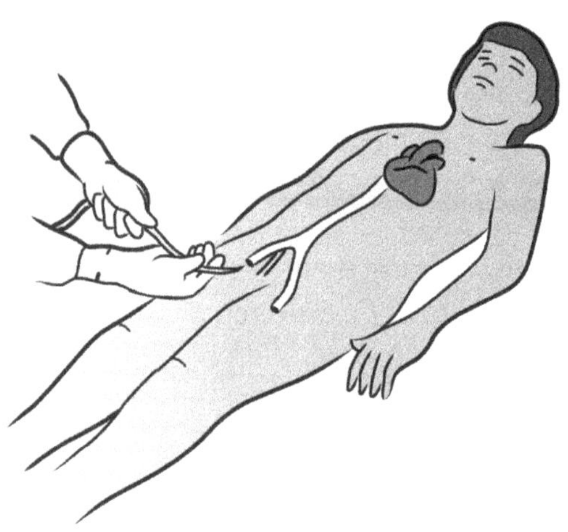

tional pillows to get comfortable, be sure to ask your nurse. You want to be as comfortable as possible and not move around during the procedure so your cardiologist can get effective pictures. You will be conscious during the procedure; however, if you feel overly anxious, you may request a mild sedative.

Once you are lying on the x-ray table, the lab staff will attach the ECG to your chest and legs, similar to an electrocardiogram, which allow your heart to be monitored during the procedure. The area of the skin where the catheters will be inserted will be washed with a sterilizing solution. Monitors (TV screens) are placed on each side of you to display your x-ray pictures during the procedure to the doctor and staff. You may be able to view some of the images; however, try not to move around to get a better view of the x-ray monitors because your heart will move, disrupting the procedure.

Your doctor will make an incision into your groin or arm so

the catheters can enter an artery. To make the incision less painful, your skin will be injected with local anesthetic. The incision is made with a small scalpel, and then a needle and a short tube called a sheath are inserted into your blood vessel. You may feel some pulling and pushing in your arm or groin but it should not be painful. If you feel any pain during the procedure, tell the medical team immediately.

Once the sheath is in place, your cardiologist will insert a long catheter following the inside of the artery all the way to your heart. Radio-opaque dye is then injected into your blood vessels. When the dye is injected, you may feel a warm sensation spreading through your body as the dye travels through your bloodstream. Many patients also experience a feeling that they have urinated—this is common, but it is only an illusion and nothing to be concerned about.

Your doctor will move the x-ray camera around and take pictures on both sides of your chest. While the pictures are being taken you will be asked to either hold your breath or take a deep breath. The entire procedure will take less than one hour.

Once the procedure is finished, your cardiologist will inform you about the results. If one or more of your arteries are blocked, your cardiologist will recommend percutaneous coronary intervention (PCI), heart bypass surgery, or medication. If your physician feels heart bypass surgery is necessary, you will be referred to a cardiovascular surgeon. If your doctor recommends a PCI (inflating a balloon with a stent in your narrowed arteries in order to break up the plaque), you will have the choice of having it performed immediately following your heart cath, so there is no break between the heart catheter procedure and PCI—or you may ask to think about your decision and end the exploratory procedure.

Overview of the Procedure:

1. *You will receive a local anesthetic injection into the skin above a blood vessel in your groin or arm.*
2. *A small incision is made through the skin and a needle is inserted into the blood vessel.*
3. *A sheath is placed into the blood vessel and a catheter is inserted into it.*
4. *The catheter is placed all the way to your coronary arteries.*
5. *Radio-opaque dye is injected into the coronary arteries.*
6. *X-ray pictures of your arteries are taken.*
7. *The artery puncture site is closed.*

Possible complications of a heart cath

- *Severe bleeding or bruising happens in about 1% of patients in the groin area.*
- *Less than 1% of patients may have an allergic reaction to the radio-opaque dye or may suffer deterioration to the function of the kidneys.*
- *In less than 1% of procedures the catheter can damage a blood vessel and cause a stroke.*
- *The risk of a stroke occurs in 7 per 10,000 patients.*
- *1% of patients suffer abnormal heartbeats during the procedure.*
- *Heart attack or death during procedure occurs in fewer than 1 in 1000 patients.*

(Based on ACC/AHA data, guidelines for coronary angiography)

DECODING YOUR DIAGNOSIS

After your heart cath, your physician should be able to tell you exactly what is wrong, how serious your heart disease is, and what treatment will be best for you. Your physician may indicate that you have one or more of the following conditions:

Plaque

Indicates you have blockage in your coronary artery. Plaques are made of cholesterol, scar tissue, and calcium.

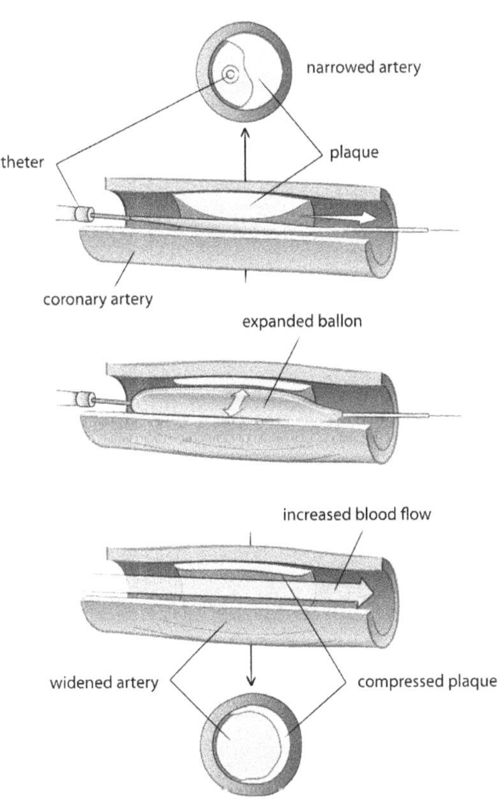

Stenosis

A narrowing in a coronary artery caused by a plaque, stenosis is classified as mild, moderate, or severe. It may also be expressed as a percentage. An artery can become 70% narrowed before symptoms of angina appear. Narrowing of 20% to 50% is a sign of early disease and is usually treated with medication and diet. Stenosis is not reversible.

Left Main Disease

This is a disease in the left (main) coronary artery, which is the most important blood vessel of the heart. If this vessel is severely diseased, bypass surgery is usually recommended, although PCI may be possible.

Occlusion

A blockage of the vessel, usually expressed as a percentage. Blockages that may have been going on for more than six months can be very difficult to unblock by angioplasty. Even if successful, the re-narrowing rate after angioplasty is high. Bypass surgery or stent placement is often recommended.

Impaired Left Ventricular Function

This means that the pumping action of the main chamber of the heart (the left ventricle) is impaired. This is usually due to a heart attack.

Heart Attack

A heart attack may be diagnosed based on symptoms, an electrocardiogram, and blood tests taken during your initial evaluation. People suffering a heart attack have certain markers in their blood that are not present in people not suffering a heart attack.

TREATMENT OPTIONS

Once your tests and procedures have confirmed that you have narrowed coronary arteries and angina, your physician will make a recommendation for the best treatment. Angina can be treated with either drug therapy, angioplasty, PCI, or coronary artery bypass surgery. Heart disease can be managed with lifestyle changes and medication.

Mild Disease

Mild disease, which is less than 50% narrowing of one, two, or three coronary arteries, is often treated with medication and diet, and it is not reversible.

Moderate Disease

In moderate disease, where 50% to 70% of the artery is blocked, treatments are determined by how serious your symptoms are and the results of other cardiac tests.

Severe Disease

Severe single vessel disease occurs when more than 70% of narrowing happens in one artery, and is usually treated with angioplasty and percutaneous coronary intervention (PCI). Severe or three-vessel disease is treated with coronary artery bypass surgery.

Drug Treatment

Whether or not they have surgery, all presenting heart disease patients will receive medication, which may include drugs for relieving angina, to reduce the risks of a heart attack, or to slow the progression of the disease. Most patients with mild to moderate heart disease are successfully treated by drug therapy alone. The more drugs you take and the higher their doses, the more likely you are to suffer drug side effects.

Percutaneous Coronary Intervention (PCI)

PCI is a procedure that involves unblocking the narrowed coronary arteries by inserting a small balloon into each artery and inflating the balloon at the site of the narrowing. This presses the blockage to the sides of the artery and stretches the arteries slightly, allowing blood to flow freely. This is similar to an angioplasty, except during a PCI, a small tube called a stent is inserted at the same time to hold the artery open. PCI is less invasive than bypass surgery because it can be performed using mild sedation and local anesthesia at the site where the catheter is inserted. A step-by-step description of the procedure will follow in Chapter 5.

Heart Bypass Surgery

If there are multiple blockages in one or more of your arteries, your doctor may recommend you undergo coronary artery bypass surgery. This is a major operation in which blood flow is routed around the clogged coronary arteries by attaching a piece of blood vessel taken from another part of the body—veins are usually from the legs, and arteries are taken from the chest wall or arm.

In other words, a coronary bypass is like being on the 10-yard line and you need to score. The defense is fired up to stop you and they call a blitz on the right side. In order to get around the defense (which is like a blocked artery), you swing around to the left side, get around the defense, and score a touchdown. The detailed play-by-play of the surgery will be laid out in Chapter 5.

Trans Myocardial Revascularization (TMR)

TMR is a procedure that is not widely used anymore. It involves boring channels in the oxygen-starved muscle using a laser, theoretically allowing blood to seep into the heart muscle from the pumping chambers of the heart. It may also stimulate the growth of new blood vessels.

Heart Valve Replacement

Heart valve replacement surgery is technically an open-heart procedure during which a damaged heart valve is removed and a new one is inserted. The new valve may be mechanical or it may come from an animal or even a human organ donor. Depending on how extensive the damage is to the valve being replaced and to your heart as a whole, you will need to be placed on a heart/

lung machine during the procedure so that the heart surgeon can stop your heart beating during the surgery. If the damage is less extensive there may be some techniques your surgeon can employ to affect the necessary repairs while your heart continues to beat.

Generally, patients who undergo traditional heart valve replacement surgery have valves that are too damaged to be repaired with a reasonable expectation of success. They must also be healthy enough to endure the stresses that the procedure and its aftermath will put on their body.

Heart Valve Repair

If the damage to your heart valve is less extensive, you may be a candidate for surgery to repair the valve rather than to replace it. In order to determine if you are a candidate for heart valve repair, your doctor will have to run a series of tests to see how extensive the damage to your heart valve is. These tests include an echocardiogram but can also include an MRI and x-rays to help your doctor form a complete picture of the nature of your heart problems.

If it is determined that the damage to your heart valve is minimal enough, your doctor may elect to do a repair as opposed to a replacement. Heart valve repair operations are generally less invasive than replacements, as your normal anatomy remains in place. Repairs allow patients to recover more quickly.

The specific technique your surgeon will use depends on exactly what type of damage has been done to the valve. For example, if the problem is a result of a floppy valve getting worse over time, the repair will involve going in and making the valve less floppy so that your valve can resume its normal function.

There is also a repair operation that can shorten the muscles and cords responsible for the opening and closing of the valves in order to restore their elasticity. The type of procedure you need will depend on the type of damage or defect on the heart valve.

Percutaneous Valve Replacement/TAVI

For those patients who need a valve replacement but who are deemed too fragile to undergo traditional valve replacement surgery, percutaneous valve replacement is a less invasive option. This procedure involves inserting a catheter through the femoral artery in the groin or a small incision under the left nipple on the chest. The prosthetic valve is then placed within the old valve and either self- or balloon-expanded to position.

While this procedure can be a better option for high-risk patients, it is still a new technology in the U.S. and is expected to have FDA approval in late 2011. This approach may not be the best choice for patients who are healthy enough to withstand a traditional valve replacement surgery, as there is no long-term data to determine success. This type of procedure is currently being done in Europe and in trial centers in the United States.

MAKING A DECISION

If the situation is an emergency, the cardiologist will proceed with the treatment that will best help you. Here are some considerations for making the best decision:

- Your health may dictate which treatment is most appropriate for you.
- Know the positives and negatives of your treatment so you can make an informed decision. This sometimes will require the input from the heart surgeon for you to make a fully informed decision.
- You may wish to obtain a second opinion from another physician.

PCI or Bypass Surgery?

PCI may be a better choice than bypass surgery if you have:

- *Suffered a recent heart attack*
- *Varicose veins*
- *Lung disease*
- *A medical condition that prevents you from having general anesthetic*
- *Suffered a stroke*
- *Kidney disease*
- *Circulation problems*
- *Already undergone a coronary bypass grafting*
- *Emphysema*

Bypass surgery may be a better choice than PCI if you have:

- *A coronary artery that has been completely blocked for an extended period of time*
- *Damaged heart valves or other conditions that require heart surgery*
- *Coronary arteries narrowed in more than one place*
- *Blockage in three coronary arteries and weakened left ventricle (decreased heart muscle function)*
- *Diabetes and more than one blocked artery*

Remember, PCI and bypass surgery can relieve your angina, but neither procedure will cure your heart disease. Even if you have a PCI or bypass surgery, you will still need to make changes to improve the health of your heart, otherwise your heart disease will continue to worsen and lead to death.

Expect the Unexpected

A Story Of Emergency Heart Surgery

Just prior to launching the new heart program in Pocatello, I had seen several patients for surgery but felt obligated to send them off 170 miles away to the customary treatment center in Salt Lake City. For many years, patients had traveled to get care in Salt Lake City, and for the most part it was excellent care, but many families had shared with me what a burden it was to have to travel, check into a hotel, and be away from home for an extended period of time. Many people had to face the quandary of deciding whether to stay home and work to pay for the medical bills or to go and be the support for their loved one. Many people would have to leave their jobs.

A patient I had seen before I had arrived in Idaho shared how he had to sell his farm to pay for his medical bills after his wife, Jean's, open-heart surgery. Jean had a heart attack and was taken by helicopter to Salt Lake City. She underwent emergency heart surgery and stayed in the hospital for more than six weeks. Her husband stayed in Salt Lake City in a motel during this time so he could be at her side.

Unfortunately, nobody was home working the farm. Jean finally made it home and recovered from a small stroke that was a complication from the surgery only to find astronomical hospital bills. She and her husband had no choice but to sell the farm. When people in rural communities have to leave homes, the burden is great on both the sick and their support team.

Within one month, our heart team would be operational in Pocatello. I now found myself scrounging to find the first patient. Dr. Ben Call, a respected third generation physician in Pocatello, sent me a patient in late November. He said, "Jake, I found the perfect first patient for surgery." The patient was Claudette Sant, a hefty 62-year-old woman who was also a brittle diabetic with sleep apnea and kidney disease. I had to stop and question, is Dr. Call my enemy or my friend?

I met Mrs. Sant in my office, and I was initially struck by her outgoing personality. She was funny and charismatic. When I asked her what she did for a living she told me that she was in charge of maintenance for an apartment building. Her daily duties included carrying refrigerators from apartment to apartment. She was a strong woman who had endured a lot in her life.

I asked her if she was married and she said, pointing to the ground, "He is down there." I immediately gave her my sympathies, as I assumed her husband had passed away, but she said to me, "It's okay, it pays well." I did not understand what she meant, and for a moment I was thinking this woman has more problems than I initially realized. She then said, "Somebody has to clean the sewers." This was the type of humor this woman had, off- key and entertaining.

After her initial work-up, I explained to Claudette the risks, benefits, and options of surgery and told her she was going to be operated on in two weeks. She told me, "Dr. Call says I am the first victim." I was a little worried starting with Claudette, as she was not the optimal candidate. A bad outcome would be disastrous for the program. She promised me, "Doctor, I'll do good, I swear!"

I had never heard of a patient promising the surgeon that they would "do good." It was reminiscent of the times when I would ask my parents if I could spend the night with my cousins, "I promise I'll be good." Not listening to my better judgment, I agreed to schedule Mrs. Sant as our first patient and put her on the calendar for December. Claudette was so excited about being the first patient she promised, "I won't let you down."

December 8th fell on a Tuesday, and I had been working for two weeks to prepare Claudette for possibly the biggest challenge of her life. Then, another message came from Dr. Ben Call telling me that he had a patient with severe coronary artery disease that needed immediate surgery. I went to meet him as he was admitted to the hospital. He was receiving an intravenous blood thinner (Heparin) and Nitroglycerin.

The patient, Ron Francis, was a good man with a positive attitude. When I met Ron and his wife, Susan, they were so thankful I was available to operate on Ron and that he would not have to travel. He told me that if he had to go away, Susan could not travel with him as she had a family member she had to care for. Tears of gratitude rolled down Susan's face when she learned that my Pocatello team and I would be available to them.

The next day I called Claudette to tell her I would have to postpone her operation. Before I could say a word, Claudette told me that she had the flu and would not be ready for surgery. The stars were aligned and we were going forward with our first operation in the new heart center.

It was late Monday evening and my team and I toured the operating room, looking over all our equipment. We went over all situations that we may find ourselves encountering. I felt like a military captain going over his strategy before invading the enemy, or like a pilot of a 747 airplane doing a walk around checking his equipment before flying. I told the team to get a good night's sleep, "It's opening day tomorrow and the ball park is sold out."

I went through the ICU and found Ron lying in bed watching TV in complete peace. Hanging from him were intravenous lines keeping his heart from hurting. I asked him how he felt and he said, "I am feeling good, Doctor." I went over everything once again with him, and then Susan joined us in the middle of our conversation. She was returning from taking care of her family member whose situation would have prevented her from traveling with her husband had he gone away for open-heart surgery.

She had such a smile on her face and kept repeating, "Thank you, thank you for everything." I told her we had done nothing yet, and she replied, "You just being here, you have done so much." I advised each of them to get a good night's rest as we had a big day lined up tomorrow. Surgery the next day was uneventful. Since ours was a new program in a brand new facility, just putting him to sleep on the breathing machine was landmark. Four days after surgery Mr. Francis went home, thankful the program was available to provide him care.

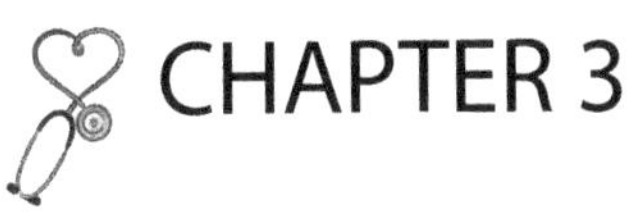

CHAPTER 3

The Team Organization

Your Doctors, Caregivers, and Cheerleaders

Just as important as having the right plays in place is making sure that your team is made up of only the best people to help you tackle your heart surgery. No team sends the same group of players onto the field regardless of the situation. Each player on the team has his own set of strengths and needs to be used in situations that play to those strengths.

Your particular condition will determine to a certain extent whom you will want to choose to make up your team. Medicine in general, and specifically cardiovascular disease, is such an extensive field that all of the medical professionals who practice in it can have very precise specializations. You want to make sure that the players you choose to make up your team are the ones most appropriate to your specific circumstances.

Specializations and skills aren't the only things you'll have to pay attention to when you're putting together your team. Any good coach will tell you that team chemistry has a huge impact on the ultimate success of any game. You need to know that the various people you choose to make up your team will be able to work well together, keep the lines of communication open, and complement each other's skill sets.

Of course, medical professionals won't be the only ones you need to have on your side throughout the process of diagnosing and treating your heart disease. Support staff and cheerleaders are vital members of your team as well, and should be chosen with the same care as you choose your cardiac surgeon.

Keeping morale up is a big part of winning football games, and it's a big part of winning the battle against heart disease, so take care to surround yourself with cheerleaders and fans who care about you, and who can keep you pumped up. Beating heart disease requires a team effort, and the better the team you can put together, the better equipped you will be to win the game.

CHOOSING YOUR SURGEON

Choosing the right heart surgeon is essential. Often your family doctor or general practitioner will make a recommendation or referral for you and there is nothing wrong with considering his or her advice. If you have a good relationship with your primary doctor it can be helpful to know which cardiac surgeon he or she would recommend for you and why. However, it is still always a good idea to do some independent research to make sure you select the right surgeon.

When you start to compare the resumes of the heart surgeons in your area, you may become overwhelmed. To make the process easier and more productive, come up with a list of important questions to ask ahead of time. Also, you can do some background research before you even meet the surgeons you are considering.

Basics

You can begin your search for a cardiac surgeon by gathering their basic information. Facts like where each surgeon did their training, how long they have been operating, and whether or not they are board certified are important things to find out. This is important because not all training programs are the same, and the duration of the training varies. In addition, a surgeon recently completing his residency may or may not have the experience that a surgeon several years in practice possesses. What about board certification? Board Certification is monitored by the American Board of Medical Specialties (ABMS). The ABMS is chartered in the development and use of standards in the ongoing evaluation and certification of physicians. ABMS is recognized as the "gold standard" in physician certification. The ABMS believes higher standards for physicians means better care for patients.

Another initial question for your potential surgeons is whether they specialize in the type of surgery you will be having. Each type of cardiac surgery is a bit different, and even though any cardiac surgeon may be capable of performing the type of procedure you need, it may not be his or her specialty.

Along these same lines, you'll want to find out how many times each surgeon has performed the type of surgery you will be having, and what kinds of results he or she has experienced. Think of this as your potential coach's personal win/loss record. You'll also want to know how many total heart surgeries each surgeon performs in a year, and even what fellow surgeons have to say about him or her.

Tips for Speaking to Doctors

Physician are used to patients' questions, so don't be shy about asking. The way the physician answers will tell you a lot about him or her.

Write out your list of questions before speaking with your doctor.

- *Ask the surgeon how many procedures he or she and their team, perform each week. You can check to see if the number compares favorably with national statistics at www.healthgrades.com.*

- *Determine if your doctor prefers to have patients on a heart/lung machine during CABG surgery or off pump and if there will be a difference.*
- *Have a good friend or family member accompany you to the consultation. Bring a notebook and pen to collect information, and even bring a tape recorder to your consultation.*
- *When obtaining a second opinion, have copies of all your test results available – even though the physician may want to run his own tests.*

** Remember, this is your life we are talking about.*

Comparing Yourself

In addition to comparing the surgeons you are considering, you will also want to find out how you compare to the majority of each surgeon's other patients. As we age, our bodies change in many subtle ways and this can have an impact on how your body responds both during and after surgery.

In addition to specializing in a particular type of surgery, cardiac surgeons can also specialize in a particular age group and co-morbid factors such as diabetes and obesity. For that reason, it's important for you to know if you fit into that specific generation that your surgeon is most used to dealing with, and if your condition is one that many of their patients have.

The Insurance Question

Another element that will have to figure into your equation when you're selecting a heart surgeon is how your surgery will be paid for and who will be responsible for the bill. You need to find out whether or not a surgeon will be covered by your insurance. You also need to know approximately how much of the bill you will be responsible for and what your options are for paying your portion.

It's important to remember that even if your surgeon is on a preferred provider list, the procedure he or she will perform may or may not be, and vice versa. As far as many insurance companies are concerned, these are separate issues so you need to make sure you receive a concrete answer to both of these questions.

Another factor that can play into the insurance element of your decision is what type of technology and technique your surgeon will use. Particularly when new or experimental technology is involved in a procedure, you will need to make sure you know exactly what your insurance company will and will not cover. For example, if you are referred for a transmyocardial revascularization (TMR) with concomitant coronary bypass operation, the insurance might only cover the bypass portion of the operation while not paying for the TMR. Be sure to check it out—you don't want any surprises that will give you heartache!

Follow-Up Care

It's easy to focus only on the details of the operation itself when you're choosing a physician to perform your cardiac surgery. However, the care you receive after can have as much, if not more, of an impact on your long-term health and prognosis as the operation itself. That's why, when you're comparing surgeons, be sure to find out what they provide in terms of follow-up care.

For instance, you will likely have to travel to the surgeon's office for follow-up visits once you have been discharged from the hospital. While the hospital where your surgery is performed might be convenient to your home, the surgeon's office may not be. It's important that you be able to get to your follow-up appointments easily.

Also, you'll want to find out what type of follow-up care and rehabilitation plan each surgeon you are considering prescribes. Some surgeons have a specific and strict course of rehab that they like their patients to follow, while others may be less specific.

The Confidence Factor

Obviously there is a lot of information you'll want to gather about each of the surgeons you are considering. However, in addition to focusing on the facts and statistics, remember to consider the human element when making your decision. You should choose a cardiac surgeon who you will be comfortable talking to and asking questions of throughout the process. This will make it much easier for both of you to share information and concerns. This will not only give you more confidence in the physician, but it will also make it easier to ensure that you receive the best possible care before, during, and after your surgery. You will likely find that once you sit down and talk with each surgeon, your decision becomes much clearer.

If you do not feel comfortable approaching your surgeon with questions or concerns, your surgeon may not receive all the relevant information about your condition and consequently not be able to provide you with the best possible care.

If you don't think you can attain that level of comfort with a younger or less experienced surgeon, even if his or her credentials are just as impressive as some of the older and more experienced surgeons you are considering, you should probably not choose that doctor, and vice versa. Your psychological preparation will have a direct impact on the outcome of your surgery and your ability to recover afterward, so be aware of your confidence level at each point along the way.

SELECTING YOUR HOSPITAL

In addition to choosing a surgeon to perform your cardiac surgery, you will also decide on a hospital where you would like to have the surgery performed. This decision will be directly linked to which physician you choose. However, the quality of the care you receive at the hospital after your surgery can have as much of an impact on the overall success of your surgery as the surgeon who performs it, so it is not a decision you should enter into lightly.

Experience

Just as it's important for your surgeon to have experience treating patients with your condition, it is also important for the hospital to have experience with patients like you. It is likely that if your surgeon specializes in the procedure you're undergoing and usually performs surgery at a particular hospital, that hospital and its staff will be well-equipped to take care of you after your surgery. It is still a good idea to gather some specific statistics.

Find out how many procedures like yours are performed at the hospital each year and how many of those are performed by your surgeon. Find out what the mortality rates are for cardiac patients at the hospital and for patients with your condition in particular. You'll also want to look into what type of training is required of the hospital staff members who will be responsible for your care after your surgery.

Also find out which hospital your surgeon prefers and why. Often the hospital where he or she operates the most will be the same one that has the most experience with your procedure. While the experience level of the hospital staff is important, you'll also want to take your surgeon's familiarity and comfort level with the facility into consideration.

Many surgeons cover different hospitals and are not based in a single institution. This is important to know, as your doctor might not come around to see you until later in the day, if not evening, and possibly not at all after surgery! Some surgeons cover hospitals across town and have commutes of up to 45 minutes between hospitals during rush hour. You will have to make the decision if this is the type of care and follow-up you want for your cardiac surgery.

Keep in mind that during an emergency, you may not have the ability to make these decisions, so be proactive and don't delay in choosing your hospital and surgeon if you have the opportunity.

Questions to Ask When Selecting a Hospital

- *Ask your physician which hospital he would choose if he was a patient, and why.*
- *Is it a city hospital with more sophisticated technology compared to a small private hospital?*
- *Is it a teaching hospital designed to benefit medical students as well as the patient?*
- *How does the hospital success rate for avoiding infection compare to the national standard?*
- *What percentage of patients have suffered a post-surgery stroke while in the care of the hospital surgical team?*
- *What complementary therapies are available?*
- *Visit www.healthgrades.com for an evaluation and ranking of the hospital where your surgeon will operate.*
- *Additional information can be found at* www.hospitalcompare.HHS.gov

Insurance

Even if the surgery itself is covered by your insurance, there may be limits on what type of post-op care it will cover. Talk to your surgeon to learn how long he or she thinks you should stay in the hospital after your surgery and then determine if your insurance covers the necessary post-op treatment. Inquire as to what the total bill will look like and how much of that will be your responsibility. Once you know this, you will be in a better position to explore alternate payment options that different hospitals offer.

Customer Reviews

There are various groups that compile information and statistics about hospitals. The specific resources available vary from state to state, but you can find out which of these groups operate in your area and obtain invaluable information from them. It's also worthwhile to find out what people who have undergone procedures similar to yours have to say about the care they received in a particular hospital.

Often there are intangible elements (the food, the view, the room's cleanliness, noisiness, or colors) that make one hospital preferable to another from a patient's point of view, and you will only be able to find this out by learning what previous patients have to say.

Types Of Hospitals

Know what type of hospital you are considering. Some hospitals are general hospitals, meaning that they are equipped to treat a wide variety of conditions and diseases. This also means that the hospital does not specialize in any one particular ailment or treatment. If your condition is a common one, a general hospital may suit your needs fine.

However, if you have a condition that is less common or if your overall health may create uncommon complications during or after your surgery, you may want to consider opting for a hospital that specializes in cardiac surgery. These specialized hospitals are generally better equipped to deal with complications and provide appropriate post-op care for patients undergoing cardiac surgery. They will also likely have access to the latest techniques and technologies available for the treatment of your condition.

Find out whether the hospital you choose is a teaching hospital. There are benefits to having your surgery in a teaching hospital. These types of facilities often have access to cutting-edge research and employ some of the foremost experts in the field. However, you should be aware that a resident may assist with, or even perform, your surgery.

Talk to your doctor about what the possible complications of your surgery could be so that you are in a better position to determine which hospital is best equipped to deal with them.

GATHERING & PREPARING *YOUR* SUPPORT TEAM

No matter how well you're able to live on your own and take care of yourself before your surgery, you'll need to put a support network in place and designate a caregiver and advocate for the period during and after the surgery. These people will become your teammates!

Your Support Team

The support team you put together can take a variety of forms. Generally it will be made up of family members and close friends who will be able to assist and support you as you prepare for the surgery and during your recovery. You may experience anxiety as you get closer to your surgery date, and the recovery process can be long and arduous; that's why it's important to have people around you that you can depend on.

For your friends and family to support you effectively, they need to know what's going on and what to expect. Take the time to notify all members of your support team of the dates and details of significant events in the course of your treatment. Also make sure they are fully informed about what you will likely be dealing with after your surgery and what may be expected of them. In fact, Chapter 8 of this book is specifically for your support team, to help them know what to expect throughout this process. A well-prepared support team will be able to serve you far better than one that lacks the necessary information.

Your Advocate

The head of your support team will be the person that you designate as your advocate throughout the surgery and immediately afterwards. You'll want to have one person who has been given authority to make decisions on your behalf and to represent your interests. Even when you're capable of making the ultimate decisions, it's a good idea to have someone with you at all of your doctor's appointments and surgical consultations both before and after the surgery.

During your appointments you will receive a lot of information, and having someone else with you to help you keep track of and ask questions about the various topics covered is a vital asset. The person you designate as your advocate may be a close friend or family member or it may be someone you hire on a professional basis. This person should be someone you trust completely to keep your best interests in mind at all times.

Exactly how much authority your advocate will have to act on your behalf is something that you can discuss ahead of time with your doctor and the advocate, and it will likely depend on your particular situation.

Your Caregiver

It can be difficult to accept assistance when you've been independent; but especially after you've had cardiac surgery it's beneficial to have help with daily activities. The person you designate as your caregiver during your recovery may be a family member, a friend, or a hired professional.

You will want to make sure that person is fully informed about what you may need help with. Give your caregiver a tour of your home prior to your surgery if he or she is unfamiliar with it so that they will know where everything is and how you like to keep things.

Also decide where you would like to spend your time during your recovery. Setting up an area for yourself ahead of time can make your transition home after surgery much less stressful for both you and your caregiver.

Multilevel Support

Undergoing any type of cardiac surgery can be a stressful process both physically and mentally. That's why it's so important for you to have a solid support network in place before your surgery. Your psychological state can have a lot to do with how quickly you're able to recover and the more emotional support you have from your friends and family, the easier it will be for you to keep a positive outlook.

UNDERSTANDING WHO IS ON YOUR MEDICAL TEAM

The following is a list of the major players on your medical team:

Physician's Assistant (PA)

As the go-between for you and your physician, the physician's assistant can help you get answers to your questions and provide information. He or she often performs physical exams and provides technical and clinical support to the attending physician. The cardiac PA is the right hand (and sometimes the left hand) of your cardiac surgeon.

Attending Cardiologist

An experienced physician who has undergone training in cardiology, the attending cardiologist is responsible for your overall care and for the decisions made by the junior staff leading up to surgery.

Blood Technician

A blood technician is trained to draw blood samples.

Cardiology Fellow

A cardiology fellow is an internal medicine physician who is trained in a specialty area such as cardiology.

Cardiology Staff Nurse

A nurse who works in the cardiology patient care unit providing patient care, the cardiology staff nurse is responsible for your well-being and safety during your stay on the ward.

Cath Lab Nurse

The cath lab nurse is experienced in the field of cardiology and may be at the monitoring station, in the recovery area, or assisting the physician performing an angioplasty. The cath lab nurse can answer your questions about the dates and times of your procedure.

Cath Lab Technician

These members of the team assist the doctor in performing the procedure by handing them equipment and documenting the procedure. They also have experience with radiology.

ECG Technician

The ECG technician performs ECGs and may also assist in other areas that require heart monitoring.

Nurse Practitioner

A nurse practitioner is a registered nurse who has advanced training and has completed a master's degree. He or she may perform physical examinations, provide patient education, and give clinical support to physicians.

Nurse Assistant

A nursing assistant undergoes training to assist nurses and provide patient care.

Resident or Intern

A resident or intern is a junior doctor in training who specialize in a particular area.

Ward Clerk or Receptionist

The ward clerk or receptionist is usually the first person you will meet when arriving at the hospital ward. He or she organizes the administration.

You might be wondering why so many people are needed to perform your heart procedure! *What happened to the old "country doctor do-it-all" model?* The truth is, we now depend on *bench strength* to win the game. Because a whopping 12% of the population is diagnosed with heart disease, we want all surgical outcomes to end positively, and we rely on specialists in all areas to accomplish this.

The Best Technician

The Importance Of Hiring A Master Craftsman To Fix Your Heart

Throughout my years of training it was ingrained in my mind that repetition leads to perfection; this statement holds true today. If you do the same thing every day you are bound to perfect it. I remember doing the same operation four to five times a day on different patients. I would leave one operating room and go to the next room and the patient was already asleep on the operating room table ready for me to make an incision. I would only ask, "Is this a man or a woman?"

I believe this type of training is an excellent model to teach the mechanics of open-heart surgery and make surgeons outstanding technicians. For example, if you owned an expensive foreign car, you would want to have it repaired by someone who was familiar with it and who worked on this type of car every day. You would not trust your expensive asset to someone who is mediocre. When dealing with your heart, you would feel the same way—you would want the best technician, a "master craftsman." However, there is a significant difference between caring for a person's car and caring for a person's body. I have never been a fan of the doctor who has his head so deep in the chest and is so focused on one aspect that he forgets what is around him.

When I was learning Radiology, the Radiologist put up an x-ray of a chest with a very large tumor in the lung. This tumor was big, the size of a baseball, in the middle of the lung. He asked, "What do you see?" The students pointed right away, one by one, to the big baseball-sized cancer in the lung. The teacher then stopped everybody and said,

"You are all wrong." He continued by asking, "If you found a twenty-dollar bill in a parking lot what would you do?" Again everybody answered, "Pick it up!" He replied, "No, I wouldn't. You're all wrong! What I would do is put my foot on it and look around, because what you got was a twenty-dollar bill, but what you missed was the hundred-dollar bill that was right next to you. In radiology it is no different. You might have seen the baseball-sized tumor, but look around because what you missed on that x-ray was another cancer on the other lung."

The point is, when dealing with heart disease, there is more to it than the technical aspect of the operation. It is the complete surgery—the preoperative preparation, the operation, and the postoperative care—that a surgeon needs to focus on. I believe that many surgeons fail to identify the entire person and the entire role of what a surgery is about.

A few years ago I took care of a heart disease patient who needed to have his aortic valve replaced. He was a retired university professor who now dedicated his days to exercising and working at the senior center. He was also very hesitant about moving forward with the much-needed surgery, as he was concerned that it would make it impossible for him to ever swim again. He was adamant about putting off the operation to fix his heart valve, but all the while the problem was getting worse and worse. We spent many months discussing the options of surgery, and I repeatedly explained to him that when he was ready I was here to help him.

It is very difficult to tell patients that they need surgery and then have to wait on them to come around; however, it is essential in dealing with patients that are sick to get them on board mentally before moving forward. I am a strong believer that, just as in basketball, baseball, or football, if the player's mind is not in the game, the game is over.

So after about eight visits and many months of talking with the patient and spending the time to mentally prepare him for surgery, he finally decided that it was time. "I am ready. I want to go to surgery," he said to me.

I immediately rearranged my calendar so I could accommodate him and prepare him for his open-heart surgery. Before his operation I held his hand, made sure he was ready, high-fived him, pumped him up, and took him to the operating room for his aortic valve replacement. His surgery went well, no problems and no complications. He was soon out of surgery and recovering in the ICU when he was faced with the uncertainty of whether he had made the right decision. Again, this is why it is imperative for a surgeon to have a **heart** when dealing with patients and not just have his or her head stuck in the chest. This was the time when my patient needed someone to reinforce his decision, hold his hand, and give him back the strength to believe he was going to recover. Prior to surgery, I had him set up a support group of friends from the senior center who were there to be with him. He went home four days post-surgery and recovered well. I saw him back a week and a half after surgery in my office. Again he needed that positive reinforcement that he would be able to swim again and get back to his activities. On his next post-surgery visit two weeks later, he was back in the pool already, doing water aerobics and feeling great!

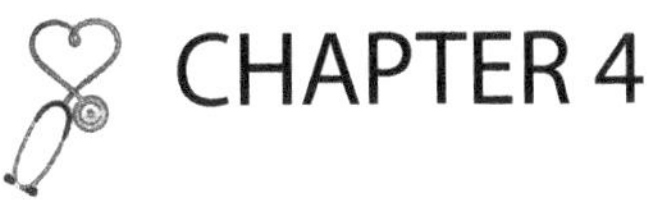

CHAPTER 4

Pre-Game Drills

Preparing For Surgery

In life, always be prepared.
Remember, all people are in pre-op.
—A.R. Moossa, M.D.

Your own personal preparation for surgery is very important to the success of the team. Your doctors, nurses, caregivers, and other team members can only do so much to help you succeed. You'll also need to make sure you're in top shape in preparation for surgery. Your psychological and physical state will have a great deal to do with how smooth and successful the outcome is.

Many athletes will tell you that pre-season training camp is the most important part of the season. If they aren't able to fully prepare their bodies and minds for the challenges of the coming season, their chances of success won't be very good. Similarly, the more fine-tuned and prepared you are prior to surgery, the greater the success of the operation and the quicker and less stressful the recovery. I work with my patients (if possible) beginning several weeks before surgery to help them prepare both mentally and physically. You can work with your doctor, or alternately, your support team of friends and family, in the same way.

CULTIVATE A POSITIVE ATTITUDE

The first thing to get in order is your state of mind. Many heart surgery patients experience a whirlwind of emotions: fear, anxiety, stress, sadness, vulnerability, resentment, suspicion, anger, and disbelief. You have the power to choose how you approach your surgery. Cultivating a positive attitude can dramatically influence the outcome.

What separates a good athlete from a great athlete? *Mental conviction combined with action.* When you believe you have what it takes to win the game, and you put those steps into place, you can achieve anything. Some people seem to be born with this innate conviction, while others develop it through experience. Still others need to be taught. If you lack the belief that you are capable of achieving anything you set your mind to, now is the time to put a new belief system into practice.

This is not about "wishful" thinking—it is about deep awareness of your true capabilities. I often tell patients: *In life, you need to have a backbone, not a wishbone.* As a health practitioner and trauma survivor, I recognize the role self-confidence and positive visualization plays in a patient's recovery. Your attitude on game day is just as important as your surgeon's skill, and it's your job to be prepared to win.

Believe you will have a positive experience. Work with your doctor, or a friend or family member, to recite daily affirmations reiterating your beliefs, such as: *I will feel great; I will be strong; My body is ready; My recovery will be swift; I have so much more life to live.*

CONFRONT AND OVERCOME FEAR

Fear is a normal experience for surgery patients. The best way to overcome fear is to confront it directly. Write your fears down (*I'm afraid there might be complications, I fear I won't heal cor-*

rectly, I don't want to die) and review them. Then write out at least ten things that you are looking forward to after surgery (*I will feel healthier than I have in a long time, I will have a better quality of life, I'll be able to play catch with my grandkids*). Now tear up your list of fears and focus on the things you are looking forward to after your operation.

MANAGE YOUR STRESS

Stress is dangerous. It places an incredible burden on your body. It can damage your health, sabotage your positive energy, and make recovery more difficult. Fortunately, there are many tools to help you manage stress effectively.

Visualization

Visualization is similar to positive thinking. It entails envisioning your desired future; for instance, being able to play a game of tennis with your significant other, waking up from your surgery feeling a renewed sense of purpose, or visualizing your blocked artery as unblocked, or your valve as working. Focus on these positive outcomes!

Healing Music

For some people, music has a healing effect. If you find music calms your spirit, whether it's Bach or The Beatles, be sure to incorporate it into your daily routine and consider having it available during your hospital stay.

Meditation & Relaxation

Many people think of the practice of meditation as sitting cross-legged on the floor and chanting "Ohm." While that is one form of meditation, there are many other ways to meditate. The goal of meditation is to distract the mind from destructive thoughts, allowing it to "let go" and embrace alternate positive and constructive thoughts.

When you return home from a long day at work, settle onto the couch, then flip the television on and watch a baseball or football game; that is a form of meditation. You may find relaxation in taking a warm bath, attending a yoga class, or getting a massage. Deep-breathing exercises can be effective, and participating in a hobby (be it working in the garden, playing a round of golf, or building a model plane) is particularly helpful for alleviating stress.

You can also listen to audio-guided meditations available specifically for people undergoing surgery, such as *Successful Surgery*, which is part of the series, *A Meditation To Promote A Successful Surgery*, by Belleruth Naparstek.

Walking

The simple act of going for a walk is an effective way to lower your blood pressure and relieve anxiety. (Note: be sure to consult your doctor before undertaking any physical activity.)

Avoid Conflict & Anger

Try to avoid intense arguments. Your health is more important than the issue that is angering or frustrating you. If you find yourself in a confrontation, take a step back and allow some time for the situation to calm down, the anger to dissipate, and the parties involved to be able to discuss the issue in a rational manner.

Get Enough Sleep

Ensuring your body receives enough rest is essential for maintaining health and avoiding stress. Here are a few ways to make sure your body gets enough sleep: avoid consuming caffeine after 4:00 pm, create and stick to a sleeping schedule by going to bed at the same time each day, get a comfortable mattress, and sleep in a cool, dark, and quiet room.

PUT YOUR AFFAIRS IN ORDER

The odds for a successful open-heart surgery are high, but it's always wise to have your affairs in order when undergoing any type of surgery. Items to consider include: updating your will (or writing one if you have not already done so), reviewing and updating trusts and beneficiaries, outlining your burial wishes, naming healthcare proxies (people who will make medical decisions on your behalf if you are unable to), appointing someone (via power-of-attorney documentation) to make decisions about your finances and property, creating a "living will," and making a list of computer passwords, safe combinations, and the locations of safety deposit box keys and important documents, such as deeds and insurance policies.

PRE-SURGERY QUESTIONS

Knowledge is empowering and comforting. Don't be intimidated to ask questions. Keep the lines of communication open with your doctor, surgeon, and other members of your medical team. The freer the flow of information between teammates in this battle, the greater your confidence level will be. Take an active role in your heart surgery planning and recovery. You are your best advocate. During appointments and consultations, carry a pen and notebook to take notes, or a recorder to record test results at your meetings, and write down questions as they arise.

Talking With Your Doctor

Learn As Much As You Can About What to Expect

- ✓ What does this pre-op test or procedure involve?
- ✓ How do you divide the sternum to get to the heart?
- ✓ How long will it take for my incision in the bone to heal?
- ✓ Will the anesthesiologist meet with me before the surgery?

- ✓ Is the anesthesiologist a fellowship-trained cardiac surgery anesthesiologist?
- ✓ What are the chances I will need a blood transfusion, and what are my blood conservation options?
- ✓ Am I at risk for anemia during my recovery?
- ✓ What are the major potential complications you will be monitoring me for?
- ✓ How much pain will I be in?
- ✓ Will I be given patient-controlled analgesia (PCA) and an IV for pain?
- ✓ How long will I remain in the ICU?
- ✓ How many of my family members will be allowed into the ICU at one time?
- ✓ How soon will I be allowed out of bed?
- ✓ When will I be able to take a shower?
- ✓ When can I drive?
- ✓ When can I have sex?
- ✓ How long should I plan to be out of work?
- ✓ How do I set up my home? Will I need to make up a room on the first floor or will I be able to climb stairs?
- ✓ Do you recommend I enroll in a cardiac rehabilitation program?
- ✓ How will post-operative pain and discomfort be managed?
- ✓ Will I be given medication for nausea?
- ✓ What are the potential side effects of the medication prescribed?

COLLECT INFORMATION FOR FOLLOW-UP

Many patients report that once they are discharged from the hospital they experience a "disconnect" from their medical team who are focused on getting patients through the surgery and the subsequent recovery in the ICU. They are not responsible for your homecare, though I can attest from my own experience returning home after my accident and rehabilitation that this is the most difficult and challenging time of the process.

In my practice, I ask my surgical patients about their home situation. I won't electively operate on anyone who doesn't have a solution and support team in place for their recovery at home. Many doctors and healthcare providers are not proactive in this area, so you may need to be.

Schedule a pre-surgery consultation with the PA or discharge cardiac nurse and ask him or her to explain to you what you should expect, both physically and mentally, once you are released from the hospital. Collect information of people you can contact for medical support, and obtain a clear directive of where and when to go for initial and subsequent follow-up appointments.

Call your doctor if:

- *Your existing symptoms become worse or more frequent.*
- *Your symptoms occur while resting or at night.*
- *Your chest pain comes on more quickly or lasts longer.*
- *You notice new symptoms, such as heart palpitations, a fast heart rate, an irregular heartbeat, or shortness of breath.*
- *You gain more than 5 lbs. in one week.*
- *You experience swelling in your ankles or hands.*

WRITTEN CONSENT

Before undergoing surgery you will be required to provide *written consent*, or permission to operate. You may be asked for consent on the day of the surgery or in a pre-admission clinic. You should have a clear understanding of what you are granting permission for; you're entitled to know why you need to have a particular procedure, what will happen during the procedure, what risks are involved with the procedure, and what alternatives are available. *You'll want to read the entire form before signing.* If you are unclear about anything, ask questions.

PRE-ADMISSION TESTS

Prior to your hospital admission, you will undergo a series of tests. They may be scheduled during your initial pre-surgery meeting with your doctor or on another day. The exact tests you will undergo will vary and are determined by your healthcare providers. These tests are necessary and important! Attending professional staff will make each of them as comfortable as possible. Some of the tests may include:

- **Anesthesia Testing:** The anesthesia team will take your full medical history and decide which anesthesia is best for you.
- **Blood Tests:** Blood tests are performed to measure red and white blood cell counts, check how your liver, kidneys, and hormone glands are working, and to note your blood sugar and cholesterol levels for post-surgery comparison. A blood sample is also taken for blood type and cross matching in the event a blood transfusion is needed.
- **X-rays:** A chest x-ray is a standard procedure to check for lung congestion, respiratory disease, or heart-chamber enlargement.
- **Electrocardiogram (ECG):** You're probably already familiar with this procedure, which is used to check how your

heart is functioning. Electrodes attached to your chest, arms, and legs are connected to a monitor that records your heart's electrical activity.

PRE-SURGERY MEDICATIONS

It is likely that your doctor will prescribe one or more cardiovascular drugs (medications that are used to treat diseases of the heart and blood vessels) for you to take prior to surgery if you're not already on them. Cardiovascular drugs consist of the following groups: nitrates, beta-blockers, calcium channel blockers, angiotensin-converting enzyme (ACE) inhibitors, anti-platelet agents, anticoagulants, lipid-lowering drugs, anti-hypertensives, diuretics, and angiotensin-II receptor antagonists (ARBs).

The three main purposes of cardiovascular drugs are:

1. To prevent or reduce the number of angina attacks you experience *(these include beta-blockers, calcium channel blockers, ACE inhibitors, and nitrates).*
2. To treat angina attacks *(this includes nitrates).*
3. To prevent the disease in your blood vessels from escalating *(these include anti-hypertensives, anti-platelet agents, anti-coagulants, and lipid-lowering drugs).*

The medications your physician will prescribe will depend on many factors, including whether you have had a heart attack, experience high blood pressure, or are suffering from another medical condition.

PRE-ADMISSION CLINIC

You will attend a pre-admission clinic, which is designed to help ensure you are prepared for your operation or procedure. During the meeting you will be advised about what you are allowed to eat or drink prior to admission, which medications to take, how to prepare your skin, and other preparation details.

PACKING FOR YOUR HOSPITAL STAY

A hospital is not a hotel (I know you may have confused the two if I didn't point this out). The hospital doesn't provide you with fluffy, warm robes, feather pillows, and little bottles of shampoo and conditioner. There are a number of items you will want to bring with you. A few items you will *not* want to bring with you to the hospital are your valuables, such as money or jewelry. After surgery your support team can bring these in. I once had a patient bring condoms to the hospital; another snuck in cigarettes and a six-pack of beer. None of these items are worth packing for your big game day.

Items to consider packing

- *Comfortable clothing (for when you are out of the ICU) such as pajamas and a robe, sweat pants, sweatshirt (that button in front not over the head), and slippers with rubber soles*
- *A pillow and pillowcase to help you sleep more comfortably*
- *Toiletries, such as a toothbrush, toothpaste, a hairbrush or comb, deodorant, razor, shaving cream, and makeup*
- *Cases and containers (labeled with your name) for dentures, hearing aids, contact lenses, and eyeglasses*
- *A list of your medications, including both prescription and non-prescription drugs, vitamins, minerals, and herbal supplements*
- *A list of your allergies*
- *A list of recent lab-tests and x-rays*
- *Contact numbers for your family and friends*
- *Eye mask or ear plugs*
- *Mp3 player, iPod, etc. for music*
- *An extra bag for additional take-home items, such as cards, gifts, and packages*
- *Simple activity items, such as magazines, books, crossword puzzles, playing cards, or knitting*

Keeping Your Focus On the Game

The Story Of A Patient Who Just Needed A Coach

In the first month I began performing heart surgery, I received a phone call from a cardiologist who wanted to send me a patient that had been turned down for surgery by the chief heart surgeon in Boise, Idaho. He mentioned that he believed I would probably turn her down also. I offered to evaluate her and give my opinion. He sent me the angiogram of the patient's heart vessels. I reviewed the films and noted the vessels were quite small, but were no different than vessels I previously operated on at Emory. I figured the decision not to operate was not due to the anatomy, but because of the patient herself.

I scheduled an appointment with the patient. When I walked into the room on the day of our meeting, I expected to encounter an obese, diabetic woman with poor protoplasm. I was surprised to find a smartly dressed, thin woman with her husband at her side. I talked with the patient, Mrs. Aslett, about her symptoms, her past medical history, and her lifestyle. I was enamored by her personality and responses, and I couldn't figure out why the doctor in Boise had refused to operate. After I examined Mrs. Aslett, I asked her why she was turned down for surgery.

She responded, "The doctor saw me in a wheelchair and assumed that I could not walk. He never asked me how I felt."

She was not in a wheelchair today, and I asked her why she had been in a wheelchair when she met with the previous doctor.

She told me, "Doctor, I was tired and I just needed a place to sit."

Her strong personality, and her desire to live and to

always succeed in what she started made her an excellent candidate for surgery. Unfortunately, I was in a quandary: the operation would be challenging, but doable; however, people would question why a physician in a new and untested program would operate on a patient when an established heart program had turned her down. And the new facility would not be ready to handle this type of operation for at least two months. I explained this to the patient and advised her that I should send her somewhere else to be operated on and stop her "heart from hurting."

"I will come back in two months. I want your hands on my heart," she replied.

I argued that she needed help now, as she was experiencing angina (chest pain).

She said, "I would rather die than not have you operate on me. You will be my coach, without you I will not get through the game."

Two months passed, and I routinely checked in with her to see how she was feeling. One week before her surgery, we began our "pre-game" drills.

I would call her and ask, "How do you feel?"

"Okay," she would respond.

"You're not okay, you're GREAT," I would yell back.

"Okay, I'm GREAT," she'd reply. We repeated that every day up until the day of surgery.

The day of surgery, as she was going to sleep, her last words as I held her hand were, "Doctor, I feel great."

One hour after surgery she was awake, sitting up looking at me with her right thumb up, mouthing the words, "I feel great." Three days later she went home with her family. Five years later, she said hello to me at a restaurant with her family. She still has a smile and is extremely thankful.

The power of the mind is incredible, and this patient was a perfect example of what someone can do if they put their mind "in the game."

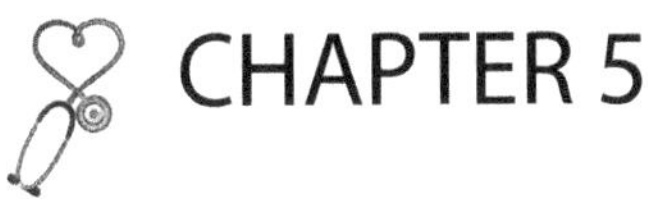

CHAPTER 5

The Big Game

Surgery

Once it's time for your surgery, your healthcare team will take over. Here's where all your pre-op preparation pays off.

You'll know that you and your team are prepared and have plays in place for the big game. The amount of time the procedure will take will depend on what type of surgery you're having and what issues arise along the way. If you familiarize yourself with the steps involved in your surgery ahead of time you'll know what to expect on the day of your procedure and what will be expected of you.

Your opening play is only one of many that will help you get to the goal line. This chapter outlines the Percutaneous Coronary Intervention (PCI) *and* heart bypass surgery procedures so you have the knowledge to start the game from a winning position.

PERCUTANEOUS CORONARY INTERVENTION (PCI)

Before your procedure you will be given blood-thinning medication to successfully prevent blood clotting either in your blood vessels or on the equipment. Blood clotting is a natural process in which platelets (tiny cell fragments in the blood) and blood proteins bind together to form a clot. Blood clots can be important lifesavers after an injury, but can be dangerous during surgery. During a PCI it is common for blood clots to form inside blood vessels, cutting off blood flow and causing a heart attack; therefore, blood-thinning medications are used.

You will also receive blood-thinning medication during your PCI. Heparin blocks the action of the blood clotting proteins and is given intravenously in combination with the oral blood-thinning medication. To ensure your blood is not overspent, a blood sample will be taken during your PCI for activated clotting time and partial thromboplastin time tests.

A guide wire, which is used to help direct equipment such as the balloons and stents into your narrowed blood vessel, is inserted into the guiding catheter and then, using an x-ray camera, its tip is carefully navigated down your blood vessel.

If your blood vessel is completely blocked, rather than just narrowed, and is more than a few months old, it may not be possible for your physician to pass a guide wire through the narrowed region of the blood vessel. Unfortunately, if this happens, your PCI procedure cannot proceed.

Once the guide wire is in place, the next step is usually to insert an angioplasty balloon along the guide wire and into your narrowed blood vessel. It is then inflated and deflated using a handheld pump. You may experience angina symptoms as the balloon is inflated.

PCI uses equipment that is slightly different from the equipment used during your heart catheter procedure. The diameters of the catheters are usually larger, and the guiding catheters are stiffer to provide extra support to the equipment.

Your interventional cardiologist will take additional x-ray photos throughout your PCI to guide him and to assess the results of the balloon inflation or stent insertion. Nitroglycerin may be injected directly into your narrowed coronary artery to help relax the artery before the pictures are taken.

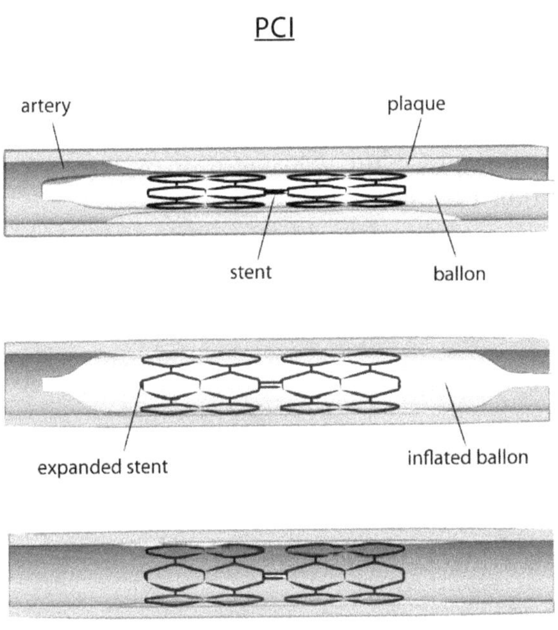

Stents are tiny tubes made of metal mesh placed at the site of the blockage to hold the walls of the blood vessel fully open. Some stents are self-expanding while others require a balloon for delivery. You should not feel the stent when it is being expanded or after the procedure is completed. The type of stent that you will receive will depend upon what is available in your hospital and which stent your physician recommends.

Closing The Incision

If you have had PCI via your groin, your physician may leave the sheath in place for 4 to 6 hours after PCI, during which time you will lie flat on your back in the recovery room. This allows time for some of your blood-thinning medication to dissipate. An alternative to sheath removal is the use of closure devices, which can reduce the time you need to spend in bed. The closure device will either plug or tie shut the hole in your leg artery. Closure devices are applied in the sterile environment of the cath lab following the PCI procedure. Closure devices allow you to move around within a few hours after surgery.

You will then be transferred to a special ward or recovery area. If you experience any pain after your PCI procedure has ended, be sure to tell your doctor.

PCI Overview

1. *You are given blood-thinning medication.*
2. *A guide wire is passed through the catheter and into the narrowed region of your coronary artery.*
3. *The PCI balloon travels along the wire into the narrowed blood vessel.*
4. *The balloon is inflated and deflated to widen the artery.*
5. *A stent is placed in the artery.*
6. *Other procedures may be performed, if required.*

Other techniques your physician may use:

- Atherectomy devices are used to remove plaque from the walls of a narrowed blood vessel before balloon angioplasty or stent insertion to make it easier for the physician to inflate the balloon completely.
- Because blood clots are common in coronary arteries and can lead to heart attack, your physician may use a thrombectomy device before inserting an angioplasty balloon and stent to reduce the risk of heart attack or other complications. These devices remove blood clots by suction.
- Drug-eluting stents (DES) may be used to help reduce the risk of re-narrowing.

CORONARY BYPASS SURGERY

Coronary bypass surgery restores blood flow to your heart by attaching, or grafting, one or more new veins or arteries onto your coronary arteries below the level of the blockage. The traditional procedure takes 3 to 4 hours.

The Step-By-Step Procedure

First, you will be taken into the operating room and placed onto the operating table. (You may notice that the room temperature is cool.) Once you are on the operating table you will be covered with a blanket and placed in a position so that both arms are outstretched. You will be attached to several monitors that allow the team to view your progress during the procedure. You will be attached to an ECG, blood pressure cuff, and a pulse oximeter (a small clip placed on your ear or finger used to measure the amount of oxygen in your blood). Two narrow tubes will be inserted into your wrist and forearm, one into a vein and one into an artery. The IV is used to deliver drugs and fluid, and the arterial line is for sampling blood and providing real time blood pressure monitoring.

Once your monitors and lines are in place, you will be given a general anesthetic. An assistant will place an oxygen mask over your mouth and nose, and you will be asked to breathe normally. The general anesthetic includes drugs to help induce sleep, to keep you asleep, and to relax your muscles.

Once you are asleep, your anesthesiologist will place a tube down your windpipe and attach it to a ventilator that will breathe for you during surgery. The anesthesiologist will then insert an additional IV line into your neck to provide access for the pulmonary artery catheter to monitor your heart pressure and activity. A bladder catheter is then inserted to drain and measure your urine during the procedure, and may be kept in for up to 48 hours after the procedure. A plastic tube called transesophageal echocardiogram (TEE) is inserted through your mouth and into your esophagus. This will allow the anesthesiologist and surgeon to evaluate the heart in real-time. Following the surgery, the TEE is removed and a plastic tube may also be inserted through your nose and/or your mouth into your stomach to prevent vomiting after you wake up from the surgery.

Once all the lines and tubes are in place, your body will be cleaned from neck to foot with an antiseptic solution and then covered with sterile drapes.

Most coronary artery bypass procedures involve making a cut down the middle of the breastbone from just below the neck to the lower part of the chest. The breastbone is then divided using a special power saw and the bleeding is controlled using an electrocautery device. The edges of the breastbone are lifted up and outward and held in place using a retractor. The protective sac around the heart is then opened to provide access to your coronary arteries.

During coronary artery bypass surgery, your blocked coronary arteries are bypassed using blood vessels from elsewhere in your body that are grafted onto your heart. Your surgeon will select the best bypass graft or conduit for each coronary artery. The blood vessels used for the bypass need to be free of disease and blockage and must match in size the artery that is being bypassed. Once the artery or vein is harvested, it is placed in a blood or heparin solution until it is needed. The incision in the arm or leg is sewn closed.

Types Of Grafts

There are three types of common bypass grafts:

- Internal thoracic artery
- Radial artery
- Leg vein

Internal Thoracic Artery Graft

The thoracic arteries run down the underside of the chest wall. They are the most common choice for bypass grafts. They have excellent long-term results, with a 95% rate of still being open ten years after surgery.

Radial Artery Graft

The radial artery runs down the forearm, parallel to the long bones. The radial artery is often used for a graft because it is long, easy to remove, and has good long-term results (an 89% rate of remaining open up to five years after surgery). Before the radial artery can be used, a test will be performed to ensure the other major artery in the arm can provide adequate blood flow to your hand. To remove the radial artery, your surgeon will make a cut along the inside of the arm just below the elbow to the wrist. A minimally invasive endoscopic approach (discussed in more detail below) can also be used.

The disadvantages of a radial artery graft are that the arm is often sore and swollen after the procedure, and in rare cases motor control may be permanently affected. You may also need to take medications for three to six months after your surgery to prevent spasm. If a radial artery graft is used, I prefer it be taken from the non-dominant hand.

Leg Vein Graft

The saphenous vein begins at the top of your foot and stops near your groin. It is usually removed through an incision the length of your leg unless a minimally invasive endoscopic approach is used. The advantage of a vein graft is that it is quick and the vein is easy to remove. The vein grafts are more common for patients more than 70 years of age or for those who need emergency bypass surgery. The disadvantage of a vein graft is it can commonly become blocked. And many patients complain of discomfort and continuous weeping from the harvesting site on their legs.

Since 2001, I have exclusively used the minimally invasive endoscopic approach for vein harvesting, and I recommend this approach for patient comfort.

The Heart/Lung Machine

Once the grafts are removed, you will be connected to a cardiopulmonary bypass machine, also known as a heart/lung machine. The heart/lung machine allows the surgeon to work on a heart that is not beating. The heart/lung machine takes over the job of oxygenating the blood and pumping it through the body. Once the heart/lung machine is implemented, the heart is stopped using a chemical solution. The bypass grafts can then be attached.

The number of bypasses you will receive during surgery depends on how many blocked arteries you have. Your surgeon will usually bypass all significantly blocked coronary arteries or regions unless they are too small. The procedure involves your surgeon making an opening in the coronary arteries just beyond the blockage, one end of the graft is affixed to the opening with sutures; the other end of the graft is connected to the aorta. Once the grafts are connected, blood is able to bypass the areas of blockage.

Once the bypasses are attached and the procedure is completed, you will be disconnected from the heart/lung machine. Your heart will be warmed, and it will begin to beat again. The amount of blood that averted into the heart/lung machine will be decreased. Once your heart is beating strongly on its own, and your blood pressure is stable, the heart/lung machine will be turned off and the ventilator will start breathing for you.

Drainage tubes will then be placed in the space between the lung and the rib cage and in front of the heart. These tubes remain in place for one or two days to drain excess fluid from the surgery site. The breastbone is closed with permanent stainless steel wires. Then the tissue above the breastbone is closed with dissolving stitches.

You will then be moved to the intensive care unit (ICU).

BEATING HEART SURGERY

Beating heart surgery involves operating on a beating heart. During the surgery the heart/lung machine is not used.

Off-Pump Surgery

The off-pump surgery procedure is the same as that of traditional bypass surgery, except the heart/lung machine is not used; instead devices are used to stabilize the area that is going to be bypassed.

The only advantages that have been demonstrated in prospective randomized studies of this method are one less day in the ICU and fewer blood transfusions.

The American Heart Association has stated that if you were trained to do beating heart surgery and you do it regularly, there is no difference in a traditional coronary bypass surgery with a heart lung machine versus off-pump.

Minimally Invasive Bypass Surgery

Minimally invasive bypass surgery, also known as keyhole heart surgery, or MIDCAB, involves performing surgery on the beating heart by making just a small incision between the ribs under the left breast and using a small camera, or direct vision, to see the heart.

The advantages of minimally invasive surgery are that a blood transfusion is less likely; no large incision is made in the middle of the chest; and patients often have a shorter stay in the ICU and usually return home within three days. The disadvantages of minimally invasive surgery are that the procedure is suitable for only a specific group of patients, and generally morbidly obese patients can be quite difficult to operate on using this method.

Coronary Bypass Surgery Overview

1. *You will be connected to monitors, such as ECG pads and a blood pressure cuff.*
2. *Plastic tubes are inserted into an artery and vein in your arm and neck, under local anesthetic.*
3. *An oxygen mask will be placed over your mouth and nose, and you will be allowed to breathe normally.*
4. *You will be given a general anesthetic through the intravenous line.*
5. *Once you are asleep, you will be attached to a ventilator.*
6. *Additional monitors and tubes will be attached to you.*
7. *You will be washed with antiseptic and covered with sterile drapes.*
8. *Your chest will be opened along the breastbone.*
9. *The vein grafts will be removed from your legs.*
10. *You will be connected to the heart/lung machine.*
11. *Your heart will be stopped and cooled.*
12. *The graft will be attached to the outside of your heart.*
13. *Your heart will be warmed and restarted.*
14. *The heart/lung machine will be turned off, and the ventilator will breathe for you.*
15. *The heart/lung tubes will be removed from your heart.*

16. *Drainage tubes are then placed in your chest to measure bleeding after the surgery.*
17. *Temporary pacemaker wires are placed on the surface of your heart and brought out through the skin.*
18. *Your breastbone is closed with permanent stainless steel wires.*
19. *The tissue above the breastbone is closed with dissolving stitches.*
20. *You will be taken from the operating room to the ICU, while you are asleep and connected to the ventilator.*

Touchdown

The Story Of A Small-Town Sheriff's Heart Surgery Recovery

Often you hear, "If I knew then what I know now, what a difference that would make." I believe this statement with all my heart. What separates the good athlete from the great athlete? Mental conviction. The belief that you can do anything, you can win anything, and you can be anything comes from the inside. Some people are born with this instinctive feeling; others develop this attitude. Some have it taught to them, while others never experience this feeling. One of my most unforgettable patients was the embodiment of positivity; from him I saw that in surgery—and in life—this attitude made all the difference.

While in the operating room one afternoon, I answered a call on my headset. I was busy sewing together two arteries using thread thinner than hair (some would call this coronary artery bypass, but I say I am giving new life to the patient).

On the other end of the phone call was my assistant Stacey, explaining that Mr. Sprague, the retired sheriff, was upstairs in my office with baseball caps for the team from Driscoll Potatoes in American Falls, Idaho. The Sheriff felt great and just wanted to let his doctor know.

Six months previously, I had performed open-heart surgery on the old Sheriff. His valve had failed him, and he also had a hole in his heart. When I first met the Sheriff he was ready to go to surgery yesterday! His mind was positive and ready to play in the game. As I had started a new heart program in a small city, many were hesitant about doing such a big operation on a high-profile individual so early in the program. What's more, many in the town were already skeptical about the idea of having heart surgery done in their hometown at all, but I knew after meeting the Sheriff, no matter what, he would do great.

When I discussed with the Sheriff his positive attitude and his winning personality, I asked him if he had always had this. He laughed and said, "No way." The Sheriff was raised in Oklahoma. Being half Native American, he grew up with negative reinforcement; being told he would dig ditches his entire life. He said one day his football coach pulled him aside and told him that he could do whatever he wanted in life—if he believed. This conversation changed his life, and from that day forward, he believed he could do anything.

Not only had the Sheriff rebounded from heart surgery, he was the longest running elected official in Idaho. He believed he could do it, and he did. I often tell patients about him because I believe that people, including myself, learn best from examples. And Sheriff Sprague was an incredible example to us all. Some of the best teachers I know teach with examples and people understand. Sadly, many people have never had an inspirational person in their life.

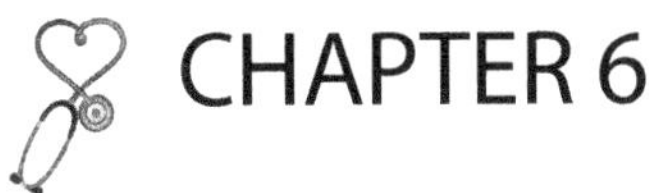

CHAPTER 6

Post-Game

Recovery

Once your surgery is over, you will move on to the next phase of your game: recovery. The time you spend in the hospital after surgery will be carefully planned out. There are many aspects of your overall health that your doctors and nurses will need to be monitoring. Each person responds differently to surgery, but you will be in a much better position if you know what you may encounter.

Just like a group of elite athletes running a series of football plays to get to that next first down, your medical team will work with you every step of the way to ensure you are able to navigate the road to recovery successfully. It's important that you have the other members of your personal team around you as well. Your family and friends will assist with your recovery.

After surgery you will spend about 24 hours in the intensive care unit before being transferred to the ward. Once you are stable and you can move around easily, you will be discharged from the hospital and allowed to go home. Most patients leave the hospital about four days after their bypass surgery.

THE INTENSIVE CARE UNIT

During your stay in the ICU a specialized medical team will be assigned to care for you. Here's what you can expect in the ICU:

- You will be connected to a ventilating machine to help you breathe. When you first wake up in the ICU, you will feel a tube in your windpipe and notice that the ventilator is inflating and deflating your chest. You will not be able to speak. As soon as you are fully awake and can breathe independently, the tube will be removed, your throat will be cleared with a suction tube, and you will be provided an oxygen mask.
- You will have a chest x-ray to confirm that all the tubes are properly inserted and in place, and that your lungs have expanded properly.
- Your temporary pacemaker wires will be attached to a pacemaker box.
- Your blood pressure will be continuously checked.
- Blood samples will be taken to measure your blood hemoglobin, clotting time, and cardiac enzymes. These tests inform your physician if you need a blood transfusion or an adjustment to your blood thinning drugs, and how your heart has reacted to the surgery.
- Chest tubes will be used to drain the extra fluid or blood from the site of the surgery so it does not pool around your heart or lungs. This fluid draining from your chest will also be recorded. The tubes will be removed as soon as the flow of fluid decreases significantly.
- A catheter is placed in your bladder to allow drainage of urine. The tube is removed after you leave the ICU.
- Most of the tubes and lines will be removed before you leave the ICU as your health progresses. When you move to the ward you will usually have just an IV line, catheter, and pacemaker wires.

THE WARD

Once you no longer require continuous monitoring or IV drugs, you will be transferred to the ward. This usually occurs 12 to 24 hours after your surgery. During the next few days you will be encouraged to get out of bed and breathe normally without your oxygen mask, and you will begin to eat solid food. You may experience tingling or a stabbing pain caused by your chest incision. If you have a leg incision, it may cause discomfort when you first begin to walk. You may also experience discomfort in your shoulder, neck, and back muscles, and may have difficulty sleeping. These symptoms are normal. It is important to understand that the chest opens like a book and the spine of the book is where the tension is, so much of the discomfort you feel will be in the back and muscle of the shoulder.

You will undergo a daily examination measuring your blood pressure, heartbeat, and the amount of oxygen in your blood. You will be monitored for fever, pain, and difficulty breathing. You will have several x-rays.

You will be provided pain management medication usually every 3 to 4 hours. If you are still experiencing discomfort despite the medication, tell your nurse. You will also be provided antibiotics to reduce the chance of an infection. You may notice increased body weight due to bloating because of the extra fluid added to your blood by the heart/lung machine during surgery. Within the first 36 to 48 hours the fluid should dissipate.

Your incision and graft site will be covered with a dry, sterile dressing for the first 24 hours after surgery. Your temporary pacemaker wires will be removed about four days after surgery. You will take your first shower 48 hours after surgery.

You will also begin an exercise plan, working out 5 to 20 minutes each day. The activity level will be gradually increased to prevent blood clots forming in your veins.

After PCI

You will be transferred to the ward for recovery. A blood sample will be taken, and you will be connected to a heart monitor that displays your heart rhythm. An ECG will be performed, and your vital signs and intravenous lines will be checked regularly. Your blood will be tested to ensure your blood count has not fallen, to check for damage to your heart, and to evaluate your kidney function.

If your PCI was performed via your groin, your physician may leave the sheath in place for a few hours after your procedure to allow the affects of the blood-thinning drugs to wear off and reduce the chances of bleeding or bruising. If the sheath is left in place, you will be kept flat on your back in bed for 4 to 6 hours before it can be removed. When your sheath is removed, pressure will be applied to the area for 15 to 30 minutes to prevent bleeding. Your physician may choose to use a closure device for your groin, which can cut the amount of time you spend in bed.

If your PCI has been performed via your wrist, the sheath is removed immediately and replaced by a small clamp or tight bandage to stop any bleeding. When this has been done, you can sit up in bed right away and your wrist will be checked regularly by your nurse for any bruising, swelling, or bleeding. The bandage on your wrist is normally removed within 1 to 2 hours and replaced with a small adhesive bandage.

Food and drink are delayed for a few hours after your PCI in case any complications develop. Once your condition is deemed stable, your family and friends will be able to visit with you. You may experience slight chest pain or discomfort, which should improve gradually within a few hours. If the discomfort becomes worse, or does not improve, be sure to inform your nurse.

You will probably only spend one night in the hospital after your PCI before being discharged. You will receive a pre-discharge consultation during which you should ask any questions about the success of your PCI, prescriptions, who to contact in case of an emergency, and how to care for your wound, along with a list of any necessary follow-up appointments.

Coughing, Deep Breathing Exercises, And Eating

You will be shown breathing exercises and coughing techniques to keep your lungs clear and help you increase the force of your breath. It is important to eat well to speed the healing of your incision and your body.

COMPLICATIONS

An irregular heartbeat is common and occurs in about one third of all patients. It usually starts on the second or third day after surgery. Your heart rhythm will be monitored and the medical team will treat it with medications. Heart attacks occur in 1 in 20 patients, and are usually mild and can be treated with medication. Kidney failure may occur in some patients who have kidney disease or diabetes—if it occurs in the hospital, it will be treated with kidney dialysis.

About 30% of patients may be disoriented, confused, speak strangely, or act oddly for a few hours or days after the surgery. Post-operative depression is common on the second or third day after surgery. About 1% of heart surgery bypass patients will experience stomach pain or ulcers—your doctor may prescribe medication to prevent these symptoms.

DISCHARGE FROM THE HOSPITAL

You will be provided information on a cardiac rehabilitation program and given a 24-hour emergency number to call in the event of any problems.

Discharge Checklist

- ✓ Review dietary requirements.
- ✓ Have your exercise physiologist demonstrate your prescribed daily workouts.
- ✓ Discuss the detailed home instruction packet with your nurse or physician's assistant.
- ✓ Ask your home care advisory nurse exactly what to expect at home.
- ✓ Have the hospital pharmacist provide both the generic and the original brand names of all medications you will be taking during recovery.
- ✓ Ask for non-childproof lids on your medicine bottles.
- ✓ Arrange to have a meal or snack available for you as you arrive home.
- ✓ Obtain emergency contact information, specifically names and phone numbers.
- ✓ Understand which medications to take when, how much, and for how long.
- ✓ Find out when you need to schedule your first post-operative appointment and if it should be with your surgeon or a local doctor.
- ✓ Determine under what circumstances you should call 911.

Playing To Win

The Story Of An Ornery 89-Year-Old Patient

In all sports, the players are loud—talking and carrying on until the coach enters the room. Good coaches inspire, make you dream, make you believe in yourself, and give you the strength to accomplish anything. There are also bad coaches that never challenge you, don't inspire, and fail to listen.

In treating people with defective hearts that need fixing, many patients have told me that they have dealt with physicians all their lives that were like bad coaches. They tell me that I inspire them to do well after surgery because I push them. I often tell patients when I meet them before surgery, "You don't really know me now, and you're going to hate me while in the hospital, but you will love me when I get you home alive." This statement is not far from the truth.

When patients first meet me, "the doctor," they don't know much about me except that I am the specialist that will operate on their heart. Immediately after surgery, I am in their face pushing them to breath, to walk, and making them believe they can do anything! I am an equal opportunity employer, no mater how old, what gender or color, I do not discriminate. I beat on everybody!

For example, I operated on an 89-year-old female from Burley, Idaho. She had a myocardial infarction (heart attack) but her ventricle was working well. The cardiologist did not do any angioplasty or stenting because she was diabetic and had multi-vessel coronary artery disease. When I went to see her, the ICU nurses and staff assumed that I would say no to surgery, and push the cardiologists to do a suboptimal procedure.

I walked in to meet her and the first words out of her mouth where, "Who the hell are you?" I knew right away that this woman would be a great patient. I introduced myself to her and her daughters, and I asked her, "Are you ornery?" She replied, "No, I am not, I just tell the truth." Her daughters immediately disagreed with a unanimous outcry, "She is ornery, and she hates men." This woman's fire in her belly, her cantankerous attitude, and yearning to fight would pull her through anything, especially surgery.

I gave her my standard lines and told her how I was going to push her after surgery like no one ever had. She responded, "Bring it on." When I told her she would love me when I got her home alive she said, "I wouldn't hold my breath if I where you."

I operated on her on a Thursday morning and did her coronary bypass surgery with the beating heart method. I chose to do her operation via this method because she was obese, elderly, diabetic, and had poor lung function. Three hours later she was back in the ICU in critical condition. She was being taken off the breathing machine, and I asked her, "Can you hear me?" She gave me no response. I asked her again, "Can you hear me?" and again no response. My sphincter was tightening; though strokes are infrequent, in this advanced age population they do occur. I asked her again, "If you can hear me, show me a finger."

This open-ended question was like asking a kid to have free reign in a candy store. I looked closely at her for a response, and her right arm started lifting. Most people lift up their thumb or right index finger, but my ornery 89-year-old gave me the bird with her middle finger and a grin on her face. At that moment, I knew she was great.

One year after her initial operation, I had the pleasure of seeing my ornery patient again at a celebration honoring the success of the heart center. She came up to me to thank me for everything I did for her. She was in tears as she gave me a hug; her daughters were behind her, also with tears in their eyes. She said, "No one has ever pushed me or made me believe in myself my entire life. If I would have met you sixty years ago, I might have done something special with my life."

The tears were now running down her face and sadness had taken over her smile. I immediately pulled her away and stopped her! I said to her, "How wrong you are." I turned her around and I told her to stop her dribbling and to open her eyes. I pointed to her four daughters, and their children, and their children's children. I told her, "You did do something special." Then the waterworks really turned on and everyone was crying.

As a physician, I believe it is my role to push and to inspire, but to also be the cheerleader. Many doctors forget what it was like to lose the big game, or to have that love of your life break up with you and leave you sad and alone. Having that special someone like your father, mother, brother, or sister come to your side and just give you a hug or pat you on the back makes all the difference in those times. Our patients need that also. We need to be strong in our conviction, but gentle in our touch.

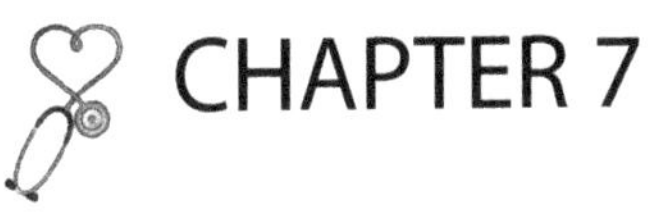

CHAPTER 7

Home Game

Recovering At Home

Like any major procedure, heart surgery places stress on your body and you will require time to recover and recuperate.

Once you're back on your home turf, completing many of your normal daily activities may be challenging. You will likely need help adjusting and working toward regaining your independence.

However, you'll have a distinct set of advantages at home that you didn't have in the hospital. Many people say they feel instantly better when they are able to leave the hospital and return to the familiarity of their own house. Surround yourself with things and people that make you comfortable and happy in your recovery.

Returning home is also a confidence booster because it helps you to feel that you're making real and concrete progress. However, it's important that you know what to expect upon your return home so that you don't become unnecessarily frustrated.

GOING HOME

You will be given a 24-hour telephone number before you leave the hospital in case you have any problems or concerns after leaving. You may arrange for someone to assist you with your home recovery, to help you take care of your wounds, and to help you with your daily activities. Being so dependent on someone else may be difficult for you, and where you choose to get that help from is an important decision in playing the game of recovery. You may want to have a close friend or family member stay with you, or you may be more comfortable accepting assistance from a home health aide hired for that specific purpose.

No matter whom you choose from among your personal team members to assist you in your transition to home life, it's important that you accept the necessity of receiving that help. You can't do this on your own any more than your surgeon can operate without his or her medical team. Your teammates are there to support you and it's your job to take full advantage of this if you want to win the game.

Preparing For Your Home Recovery

- *Determine which items should be moved so you do not have to reach your arms up for anything heavy, such as items in the kitchen.*
- *Consider preparing meals ahead and freezing them for your return home.*
- *Designate and set up a cozy recovery area.*
- *Prepare an area to keep your medications and your medication chart.*
- *Decide where you will take your daily walks.*
- *Select a location where you will perform your daily exercises.*

Visitors

Visitors may cause exhaustion, so it is important to pace your daily routine accordingly; limit the time you spend on phone calls, answering e-mail, and visiting with friends and loved ones.

Call Your Doctor if:

- *You have a fever greater than 101°.*
- *You experience excessive drainage that is red.*
- *You have redness, swelling, or pain at the site of your incisions.*
- *If you gain five pounds within one week.*
- *If you experience severe pain in your chest, back, or shoulders.*
- *If your heart beats rapidly or skips a beat when you are resting.*

If you experience pain or breathlessness...

* It is not normal to experience breathlessness, central chest pain, or pain radiating down your arms. If you experience this, call 911.

YOUR HOME TEAM

Your primary caregiver may be your spouse or partner, a friend, or another family member who can help you with regular household tasks, as well as with your recovery by being your nursing aide, providing transportation, and coordinating your medical care. However, it may be difficult for your primary caregiver to be on-call 24/7. That's why it's a good idea to set up an expanded home team.

Here's how your team can help you:

✓ Prepare nightly dinner.
✓ Provide practical advice.
✓ Provide emotional support.
✓ Run errands, such as to the supermarket, to the pharmacy, and the laundry and dry cleaner.
✓ Do the housekeeping.
✓ Chauffer you to your rehab program and social events. (Be aware that it will be 4 to 6 weeks before you will be able to drive a car.)

CARING FOR YOUR INCISION

Gently wash your wound every day with a washcloth, mild soap, and warm water while you're in the shower, and pat dry with a towel. Do not put ointments, creams, or moisturizers on the incision. Check for any drainage, redness, or swelling, or any signs of infection (such as feeling hot at the site of the incision).

Tips for Managing Pain and Discomfort:

- *Wear loose clothing.*
- *Take your pain medication as directed.*
- *When you cough, place a pillow to your chest.*
- *Drink 6 to 8 glasses of water per day, unless otherwise instructed by your doctor.*

Chest Wound

The wound is epithelialized (waterproof) in 24 to 48 hours, and takes 4 to 6 weeks to heal. Complete healing of the wound takes close to one year. The chest bone will be tender, so wear loose clothing such as shirts made of soft fabric with buttons in front; not pullovers.

Graft Wound Sites

Elevating your arm or leg for 15 to 20 minutes helps reduce any swelling you may experience. If your graft was taken from your lower leg, avoid crossing your legs while sitting and consider wearing below-the-knee support or stockings to prevent fluid from accumulating.

Follow-Up Medical Visits

You will meet with your primary care physician 1 to 2 weeks after your procedure. You will also meet with your cardiologist and surgeon to have your groin or wrist examined, check your general well-being, and refill any necessary prescriptions. Depending on your status, you may meet with your primary care physician and cardiologists over the next few months for blood or exercise tests.

Know Your Medications

- *Both the generic and brand-name*
- *How much to take*
- *When and how to take it*
- *What it does*
- *Possible side effects*
- *What to do if you forget to take a pill*

WHAT TO EXPECT ON YOUR ROAD TO RECOVERY

If you had a heart cath or PCI via your groin, avoid strenuous exercise and heavy lifting for 1 to 2 weeks. If you had a procedure via your wrist, avoid activities that may put a strain on your wrist, such as tennis, golf, or typing.

You may return to driving within 1 to 3 days of your cath or PCI procedure. You should be able to return to work fairly soon unless your job entails strenuous activity or heavy lifting, in which case you should wait 10 full days before going back to work.

Sleeping

Difficulty sleeping or insomnia is common after open-heart surgery. This should dissipate after a few weeks. To help with sleep, try to:

- Avoid caffeine and alcohol.
- Go to bed every night at the same time.
- Take your pain medication or sleep medication before going to bed.

Driving & Flying

You should avoid driving for 4 to 6 weeks after open-heart surgery. Medications may make you drowsy, and sudden stops while driving can upset the healing process. However, you may ride in a car as a passenger. If you plan to take a long journey it's important that every hour you walk around for a few minutes to allow your blood to circulate and prevent a deep vein thrombosis.

Eating & Drinking

Your appetite may take a few weeks to return to normal. It's important to continue to maintain a well-balanced nutritious diet even though you may not be hungry. Drink plenty of water every day, unless your doctor advises you to restrict fluids. I recommend multiple small meals instead of three large meals.

Sexual Activity

Your sexual drive may also decrease after heart surgery, but this is not permanent. You will gradually return to your normal level of sexual activity. If you experience a rapid heartbeat, have difficulty breathing for 20 to 30 minutes after intercourse, experience angina, or feel tired the next day, it's an indication to slow the pace down.

Physical Activity During The First Eight Weeks

When working out, check your heart rate during exercise. Your workout heart rate should be at least 10 beats per minute higher than your resting heart rate, but no higher than 120. Your pulse should return to its resting rate within 15 minutes of finishing your workout. If you are unable to talk while exercising, your physical activity level is too high. To check your heart rate, locate your pulse in your neck or wrist, and count the pulses for exactly 6 seconds, then add a zero. For example, 8 pulses in 6 seconds indicate a heart rate of 80.

During the initial eight weeks DO NOT:

✓ *Push, pull, or reach with your arms*
✓ *Resume household chores until the fourth or fifth week*
✓ *Lift heavy items*
✓ *Eat unhealthy foods*
✓ *Partake in a strenuous workout*
✓ *Continue to smoke*

Home Plan

DAY 1 – 2

Rest as much as possible.

WEEK 1

During the first week, gradually increase your level of activity:

- *Climb stairs slowly.*
- *Take short walks.*
- *Do the breathing, arm, and leg exercises shown to you in the hospital.*

WEEK 2 – 3

Begin to increase your activity level:
Lift and carry light objects that weigh less than 10 pounds.
Increase the distance you walk.

WEEK 4 – 5

- *Continue the breathing, arm, and leg exercises.*
- *Increase your walks to at least 30 minutes per day.*
- *You may begin doing chores.*
- *Discuss returning to work with your doctors.*

WEEK 6 – 8

You should be able to gradually resume all the activities that you did before your surgery and return to work full time.

Questions to Ask About Cardiac Rehab

- *Which cardiac rehab program do you recommend?*
- *What do you like about this particular program?*
- *What educational programs are offered aside from exercise training?*
- *How long does this program last?*
- *What does the program cost?*
- *Is the cost covered by my insurance?*
- *Is the program certified?*

Cardiac Rehabilitation

Cardiac rehabilitation is a support program to help heart surgery patients return to an active, normal life. Most patients begin a program two weeks after surgery with a referral by their doctor.

Attending a cardiac rehab program is one of the best things you can do for your recovery. It usually involves classes that last for several months and a custom-designed exercise and lifestyle program fit for your specific needs. The best thing about a cardiac rehab program is the support you receive from other heart patients.

Joining a cardiac rehabilitation program will improve your health and increase your exercise capacity. It can:

✓ Increase your mobility
✓ Decrease angina
✓ Raise your HDL cholesterol levels
✓ Improve your body's ability to use oxygen
✓ Speed your recovery
✓ Decrease the likelihood that you will have a heart attack
✓ Provide encouragement
✓ Lesson depression
✓ Reduce risk
✓ Lessen pain

✓ Make everyday activities easier to perform
✓ Improve your strength
✓ Provide a better quality of life

Cardiac rehabilitation is typically a 12-week outpatient program that you will attend three times a week for an hour each session. Each session usually includes a 30-minute exercise regimen that is monitored by an ECG. You will also learn healthy eating habits, stress management techniques, how to modify your risk factors, and about the medications you are taking.

The 30-minute exercise session is created specifically to your individual needs and you will progress at your own rate within safe limits for your condition.

How the exercise session works:

- ECG electrodes are applied so your heart can be monitored during each exercise.
- Each session begins with stretching and easy movement to warm up your muscles, prevent injury, and allow your nurse to record your resting blood pressure and heart rate before starting more rigorous exercise.
- Your 30-minute routine may include a series of short sessions using various machines, such as treadmills, stationary bicycles, stair climber, or elliptical machines—or it may focus on only one exercise method.
- As you exercise, your heart rate, heart rhythm, and peak blood pressure are monitored. Your nurse attendant will ask you to estimate your exertion level based on a graduated scale of difficulty. Gradually over the course of your rehabilitation, your activity will increase and become easier. You should notice improvement within 3 to 4 weeks of training.
- After your session you will spend about 10 minutes cooling down, stretching, and relaxing the muscles.

Not Everything Is As It Seems

The Curious Case Of A 56-Year-Old Biker Patient

Doctors are no different than society in general, we come to conclusions quickly and we size up situations before we have all the facts. Through experience I have opened my mind to reserve judgment until I have all the information because sometimes things are not always as they seem. I have seen so many physicians come to conclusions about a patient right when they walk into the room and never divert from their initial judgment. As health care providers, we must open our minds and our hearts to everyone we see in order to give the "best medicine."

Two months into doing open-heart surgery in Idaho, I experienced a situation that was not what it seemed. One afternoon I was called to see a patient in the Cardiac Catheterization Recovery Room. Dr. Fernando Grigera, the interventional cardiologist, told me he had a 56-year-old diabetic "biker" with severe three-vessel coronary artery disease. I reviewed the film with him and concurred with his assessment. Dr. Grigera told me that the man had this same disease one year ago and that it had only gotten worse. I asked why nothing had been done for this man one year ago, and I was told he refused surgery. I know most sane people would not refuse what the doctor recommends if it could save their life, but I am always surprised by what some people think and do.

I met the patient, John Maher, sitting upright on his bed. He was a forceful mouth-breather because he had broken his nose in fights in the past and could not breath through his nose anymore. As I mentioned, he was sitting up after having his heart catheterization, and anyone who has gone through this ordeal knows you have to lay flat in bed for at least three hours. He was just 20 minutes out from his procedure but he was fighting the system—as he had his entire life.

I introduced myself to him and shook his hand. He grabbed my right hand so tightly that he almost put me on disability. Out of his mouth in an East Coast, Brooklyn-type accent with nasal undertones came, "Put 'er there, Doc."

We started talking. Well, let me rephrase, he started talking. I was listening. He recounted me his entire history and also told me that he knew he should have had surgery last year when he first started having chest pain, but his wife died unexpectedly of cancer at the time he was planning surgery. He explained, "It's been a little over a year since her death, and Doc, I still think of her and miss her everyday." It turns out this tough old biker who had pushed society's rules all his life actually had a heart that was hurting in more than one way. I reached out to him, put my hand on his shoulder, and just stood with him.

I explained to Mr. Maher that he would need surgery and we needed to do it sooner than later. He agreed, and I scheduled him the next day for open-heart surgery. I spoke to his daughter and I explained everything to her in regards to her father's hurting heart. She implored me, "Dr. DeLaRosa, please take care of him, he is all I have now."

I took Mr. Maher to surgery and was planning to start operating at 7:30 am sharp. (Dr. Joseph Brown, the Cardiac Anesthesiologist, runs a tight ship and always gets started on time.) But as I walked into the operating room, Mr. Maher was laying on the operating room table not ready for surgery. I noticed there was a commotion going on at his right hand. He had a ring from his wife that he had placed on his little finger after her death. The ring had not been taken off since then. Many times patients come to surgery with rings on their fingers, in their belly buttons, or in every other orifice imaginable that cannot be removed. Unfortunately, we still need to cut them off. This is done because the metal on the body can be a conductor with the electrocautery and can burn the patient. Also, as the patient swells up after surgery, the finger can lose its circulation.

We routinely cut rings off with a metal cutter, but we try all sorts of techniques (soaping, oiling, and greasing the finger) before we resort to cutting. We tried everything imaginable with Mr. Maher's beloved ring—even tying a string around his finger to pull off the ring, but nothing worked. We finally decided after one hour of exhausting all methods and attempts that we had to cut the ring in order to proceed. We placed the metal cutter around the ring and tried to squeeze it together, but the ring would not cut. It was like the ring wanted to stay and not be removed from Mr. Maher. Unfortunately, that was not an option on this day.

I was ready to give up when I called out to our perfusionist, Mike, to come assist. Mike is a part-time body builder/naturalist when he is not saving lives working the heart/lung machine as a perfusionist. I asked Mike if he could lend his strength to cut the ring. Mike said, "First, I have to pump up." Mike started doing pushups on the floor and pumping up. Then he grasped the metal cutters and squeezed so tight his hands turned red and his eyes were popping out of his sockets. All of a sudden there was a SNAP, and for a second I thought that Mike, with all his might, snapped Mr. Maher's finger off! Fortunately, it was the ring.

Finally we got the operation underway. We did a quadruple bypass and kept the heart beating. He did well through surgery, and post-operatively Mr. Maher was without pain and progressing well. His postoperative course was benign and he went home on postoperative day number three.

One week later Mr. Maher returned to see me. He complained of feeling weak, as though he did not have any fire inside. I gave him a pep talk and told him he was great to try and snap him out of his negative thoughts. He thanked me and went on his way.

Another two months went by and Mr. Maher's daughter called me and told me her dad was not getting out of bed, was depressed, and was nothing like himself. She did not know whom else to call, so she called me. We both concluded that he must be depressed. I told her to bring him in again so we could snap him out of his depression.

When I saw Mr. Maher, he looked like a Mack truck had hit him. He was disheveled and miserable looking. I talked to him and tried to inspire him, as his daughter did also. He said, "Doctor, my legs are weak, and I have no energy to even get up in the morning. I really want to try but I just don't feel like it."

I told him that if he did not snap out of his depression he would end up in a nursing home or even a psych ward. His response to me was, "Okay, I guess you are going to have to do that." I was so sad to see the strong "biker" become so weak and unable to arm a fight. For a moment, I thought of the ring I cut before surgery—perhaps it had given him strength before and now I had taken it away.

Mr. Maher's daughter sat in the exam room crying, listening to her father give up. She cried out, "Damn it, I need you!" I explained to both of them that I wanted to rule out something organic like a stroke, tumor, or a brain bleed with the CT scan, but sadly, this was most likely severe depression and he would need to visit a psychiatrist.

The CT scan of his head was normal, and Mr. Maher saw a psychiatrist. I received a phone call one week later informing me that Mr. Maher had been committed by his psychiatrist. I was so sad, as I felt responsible for failing as his coach. What I have learned is that true mentors, role models, and leaders take responsibility when someone from their team fails, and that is exactly how I felt.

Four days later I was in my office when my assistant informed me that Mr. John Maher was on the telephone and wanted to talk to me. I thought he was committed, and I was trying to think how he got to a phone—did he escape? As I answered the phone, I heard a ruckus of noise, music, and laughter. I said, "Hello, hello?" I heard a voice, "Hello, Doc!" That nasal Brooklyn voice that I learned to miss was now on the other end of the line. I said, "Mr. Maher, are you okay?" Mr. Maher replied in his most eloquent way, "I am f'ing great, Doc!" I asked him what happened and he explained, "Ya, I was in the loony bin, but some resident doctor checked my blood for something called cortisol."

Cortisol is a major circulatory hormone in the human body that is needed for everyday use. When Mr. Maher's cortisol level came back, it was so low that the laboratory had to re-check to be sure. The young doctor treated his low cortisol level with steroids, and the re-emergence Mr. Maher experienced was a catharsis. One week earlier he was too tired to get out of bed, even to go to the bathroom. He now was on his Harley, living large, and feeling great.

My experience with Mr. Maher solidified, once again, that not everything is what it seems. It is important for health care providers to listen to and understand their patients. Through the efforts of a young physician, Mr. Maher had a very curative problem that might have been over looked if not for the open mind found in a neophyte doctor.

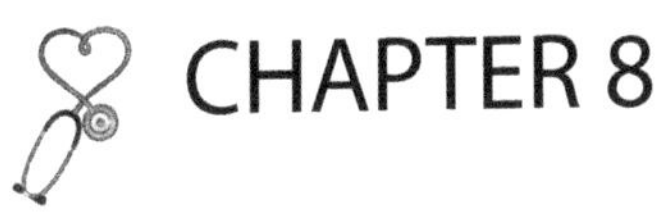

CHAPTER 8

A Word To The Team

Supporting Your Loved One Throughout Surgery

In football, your team can lead you to the goal line, lead you to the championship, or it can fail you. When your loved one is facing major heart surgery, you need to be the kind of teammate they can depend on. Your role as a member of their support team will significantly influence whether or not they have a successful outcome in the surgery game.

As a brother, sister, child, parent, neighbor or close friend, you face a major challenge when a significant other gets hurt or needs major surgery. This is almost as painful, and sometimes more so, than if you were to experience it yourself. Just as the patient undergoing surgery has to be prepared mentally and physically to have a major heart procedure, so do you, as part of his or her support team. The purpose of this chapter is to help you know exactly what to do and how to do it when it comes to being a supporting player on the receiving end of heart surgery.

Providing Support

When the patient is diagnosed with heart disease and is told the terrible news that they will have to undergo open-heart surgery or a PCI, this is very traumatizing, not just to that person, but also to you who love him or her.

When the news arrives, you immediately have to be supportive to the patient. It is your job to block for the quarterback, so to speak; though you may feel like succumbing to the hit, your job is to stay strong and offer as much support and protection as you can. Many patients will break out in tears. Others may get angry. At this traumatic moment, you must be there to offer strength, love, and the reassurance that everything will work out in the end.

Planning For The Big Game

Once the initial shock of the news has worn off and the surgery has been scheduled, it is time for the support team to mobilize for action. It is important to be cognizant of the times the patient will need to go to their preoperative appointments. This is when you will be crucial as a teammate with whom they can discuss the operation, the risks, the benefits, and the options before them. You should also be aware of the time the patient needs to be at the hospital on the day of surgery. If it is determined that the surgery will be a first case surgery, this could mean an arrival to the hospital as early as 5 am. It is important to set your alarm so you will be able to transport the patient on time.

The Waiting Game

On the day of surgery, it is important for you to be as comfortable as possible. This is going to be a long day for the patient as well as you! Once the patient arrives into the pre-operative area, you will be sent to a waiting area to—you guessed it—*wait*. In my practice I like to let the support team see the patient before he or she actually has to go back to the operating room, which could be as much as an hour and a half beyond when they initially arrive. I also like to update the family on the progress of the operation, from when the incision is made and the patient goes on the heart and lung machine (if they have to), to when the repair is being done, when the patient is off the heart and lung machine, when we are closing the incision, and when we are leaving the room. I believe it is vital to update the support team/family during this time, as operations as well as procedures can last several hours.

During this time the support team can be updating other people in the support tree, filtering the information out. I believe it is important for the support team to be made aware of what is going on in the operating room; however, there are many doctors that do not like to update the family in the midst of the operation and feel that it is best to wait until he or she is out of the operating room before updating the family. If this is the situation you face, be prepared to exercise patience.

Once the operation is finished, the doctor will come and talk to you and explain exactly what they found, exactly what they did, and what can be expected.

Post-Surgery Procedure

Following the post-surgery visit from the surgeon, you and the other members of the support team will be allowed to visit the patient in the intensive care unit for a brief period. In the intensive care unit the patient will have a breathing tube, IV lines, and catheters coming out of his or her private parts and chest, in addition to all sorts of other tubes and wires everywhere. The nursing staff in the intensive care unit should cover this up, but it can still be shocking for you to see the person you love in this situation. I feel this time is very important for the patient; he or she will most likely be asleep, but they feel the aura, the vibe that is in that room.

Suffering through my accident and being in the intensive care unit for several weeks, I know that a positive thought begets positive thinking. So keep your words and thoughts hopeful during this initial visit with your loved one. This visit usually will last 5 to 10 minutes, then the intensive care unit nurses will need to get back to their resuscitation and care of the patient.

Staying In Contact

Following the visit, once again it is important for you to relay information to the rest of the support team tree. Remember to leave your and all support members' contact information, such as cell phone numbers, home phone numbers, or any other mode of contact with the nurses in the intensive care unit as well as the ward clerk. This is imperative, as the information that was given earlier in the morning can get misplaced.

I once had a patient's family leave several names to be contacted. That evening I tried to contact the family, and as I called the first number that was listed, and they responded that they would be there right away. I later found out that this person was an estranged family member who was not to be contacted for any issues or for any matters concerning the patient and did not even live in the area. Other times, the phone numbers that were listed were either disconnected or no longer in service. The doctors and nurses at the hospital must be able to reach you, so double check that the information you provide for them is accurate and reliable.

Visits From The Fans

In the days following surgery, the patient's recovery should be uneventful. It is important to limit visits, especially if the patient remains in the intensive care unit for several days. Occasionally, the support team feels it is important to bring children, grandchildren, or great-grandchildren to see the patient. *Please know that it is not healthy to bring small children into a hospital, especially newborn babies.* Many intensive care units, and my own in particular, do not allow babies under two years old to enter. Though you may not like this rule, keep in mind that patients who have recently undergone such a traumatic procedure usually will not remember whom they have or have not seen, as they are under heavy medications during their intensive care unit stay.

Once the patient is healthy enough, he or she will be transferred out to the ward/floor. Patients usually stay one or two days on the ward/floor before being discharged home; however, during this time you should still limit the number of visitors. Patients often feel that they have to entertain guests who come to visit them, and this can be very draining emotionally and physically. I routinely limit the number of visitors that can visit a patient post-surgery.

I have some patients that have large support teams and families numbering several dozen that want to come and visit, take a peek, touch the patient, and make sure he or she is alive. I understand the concern of these family members and friends, but this is a time when relaying the progress to everyone else may be more helpful than having everyone come and see the progress for themselves.

It is especially important to be aware that if a member of the support team is sick, it is not the time to be in the hospital, especially not around the patient. Hold off on the need to see the patient at this critical time, as he or she is immune-suppressed and could catch something very quickly. If a member of the support team absolutely has to see the patient, they must use good hygiene, wash their hands, and wear a mask to protect the patient as well as the other patients in the hospital.

Educating The Team

During their time on the ward/floor, the patient will be educated about what diet to follow, how to get out of bed or a chair, and how to walk upstairs. As a member of the support team, it is critical for you to be a part of these lessons and discussions. I recommend that you make a schedule with the nursing staff of when the physical therapist, dietician, and nurse coordinator will come around to discuss these issues so you can plan to be there. Though your work schedule and other demands on your time may make it difficult to always make these meetings, you can arrange with the head nurse to get you educated and up to speed on what you need to know so you will be able to provide the patient with the best care.

Ensuring The Home Field Advantage

When planning the patient's discharge from the hospital, I address a number of issues: where will they go after surgery? Who will be at home with them? Do they live alone? Do they have a support team in place at home? Do they need to go to rehab? Do they need to go to a skilled nursing home? I think it is imperative that you as a member of the support team be a part of this discussion, which I usually hold in conjunction with planning the operation.

You need to be aware of what will happen once the patient is discharged at least 48 hours prior to the event. Be involved in these discussions so you can prepare the home, prepare the medications that will be needed, and so you can make arrangements to get time off from work or school. During the discharge, talk with the nurse, the physicians assistant, and the physician about follow-up appointments, questions you may have about the medications (both old and new), how to maintain the wound, and who to contact when issues arise. It can be extremely stressful if you need to speak to somebody and you can't get through or don't know who to contact.

When you arrive home with the patient, make sure the home is already prepared for them. From my own personal tragedy I realize how significant the first days home after a lengthy hospitalization can be. In fact, I do not allow any of my patients to be home alone after open-heart surgery. It is important to have support available around the clock during this time, as complications do arise.

Sleeping

I recommend that patients sleep in a reclining chair in order to get up easier if they find their bed to be cumbersome. Don't take it personally if your loved one does not want to sleep in the same bed with you—it can be very difficult for them to have you turning or jostling next to them after having just undergone surgery. In some cases, you may request that the doctor orders a medical bed for the home; however, I do not feel this is necessary for the majority of patients. I believe patients should be discharged from the hospital only once they can take steps, get out of bed, use the toilet, shower, and brush their teeth by themselves.

Eating

At home, patients will not be hungry. Again, don't take this personally if your loved one does not want to eat the usual stack of pancakes, two eggs, three sides of bacon and toast that they were able to eat before surgery. Post-surgery patients will not want to eat big meals. Instead, the usual breakfast, lunch, and dinner menu will be divided into smaller portions, such as breakfast, mid-morning snack, lunch, late afternoon snack, dinner, and sometimes a late evening snack, in order to keep up with nutrition and keep up with what the patient needs to eat.

One Difficult Issue

The final issue to be aware of following surgery is the dreaded constipation. Patients that have just had their chest cut open especially do not want to have to push while sitting on a toilet. Many patients will be discharged with a stool softener or something to help their bowels function. In my practice nobody goes home without first having a bowel movement in the hospital. I often recommend eating fruits such as cherries and sundried prunes instead of taking stool softeners. Constipation can be a miserable, drawn-out experience that is, unfortunately, part of the recovery process. I warn patients before surgery of this as well as upon discharge.

Huddle Up!

You, as a member of your loved one's support team, are a critical part of his or her success. Remember that this ordeal is something you will experience *with* your loved one. Be a proactive part of the planning process and be a supportive and dependable part of the healing process as well. Be a team player and everyone wins!

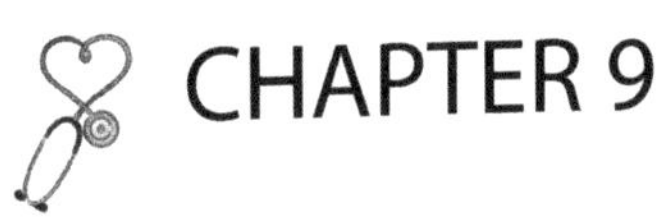

CHAPTER 9

"First And Goal On The Three"

Diet & Nutrition

As your recovery progresses and you near the goal line, you can begin to shift your focus from your immediate recovery to your long-term goals. When you're first attempting to tackle the prospect of recovering from heart surgery, you can become overwhelmed by the enormity of the challenges in front of you.

Similar to a team starting on the opposition's two-yard line, you'll need to realize that you can't cover the whole field and score a touchdown in one play. Instead you'll focus on taking one small step after another—gaining a few yards here and a couple more there, as you slowly work your way down the field.

Your road to recovery will be full of many small victories rather than one dramatic leap to the goal. As you get closer to your goal line, however, it's important that you start to shift your focus to the big picture. Your life after heart surgery must feel and be improved, not the same. There are a number of important steps you should take in order to make sure you don't wind up right back where you started health-wise.

One big part of putting together a healthy lifestyle after surgery is making a habit of proper diet and nutrition as well as exercise. For some people this will not require huge changes, but for others it can mean an entire overhaul of their eating and exercising habits. Just as with all of the other aspects of your game plan and after surgery, your success in adjusting to a healthy lifestyle will require having the appropriate team members in place and the right attitude on your part. Only you can make the decision to be healthy, but there are many people who can help you make that decision a reality.

EASY CHANGES YOU CAN MAKE TO YOUR DIET

Let's start with some easy changes you can make to your diet:

- Reduce sodium intake to less than 1500 mg per day, as diets high in sodium increase the risk of high blood pressure.
- Avoid processed foods.
- Read labels of food items to make healthy selections.
- Use low-fat condiments, such as balsamic vinegar, mustard, pickle relish, horseradish, and lemon juice.
- Avoid dressings and sauces high in fat and sodium.
- Drink healthy beverages, and eliminate soda from your diet.
- Reduce consumption of sugars.
- Eat foods high in phytochemicals, which protect against cardiovascular disease. These include: strawberries, raspberries, pomegranate, apples, grapes, walnuts, red wine, non-alcoholic grape juice, eggplant, green tea, white tea, black tea, lentils, black eyed peas, citrus fruits, pears, cherries, kale, tomatoes, potatoes, onions, leeks, broccoli, endive, chives, red cabbage, radishes, apricots, rhubarb, parsley, buckwheat, soy beans, hummus, almonds, olive oil, brussel sprouts, whole wheat, seeds, nuts, canola oil, ground flaxseed, kidney, fish Omega-3s, navy beans, pinto beans, plums, asparagus, beets, bell peppers, carrots, cauliflower, snow peas, squash, sweet potatoes, and turnips.

Foods to include for healthier eating:

- ✓ *Whole grains: including pasta, bread, and rice choices*
- ✓ *Beans: such as hummus, lentils, and black beans*
- ✓ *Fruits and vegetables (strive for nine servings each day)*
- ✓ *Extra virgin olive oil as a prime source of fat*
- ✓ *Fish: grilled, broiled, or roasted without heavy sauce or butter (strive for at least two meals per week)*
- ✓ *Nuts: eat a handful each day*
- ✓ *Chicken: roasted or grilled*
- ✓ *Herbs and spices: use as flavorings instead of salt*

KEEP A FOOD JOURNAL

Keeping a food diary can encourage you to eat fewer calories and lose weight. Keeping track of what you eat on a daily basis increases your awareness of what, how much, when, and why you were eating, and helps cut down on snacking. Keep a notebook with the following information: time, food, amount/portion size, level of hunger, location of meal, and the emotion before, during, and after eating. Each week, review your information to determine patterns that are keeping you from improving your health and finding alternatives.

EXERCISES

Here are three heart-healthy exercises to help get you started with a workout routine.

Checklist:

- ✓ Your exercise location should be safe, clean, and free of clutter.
- ✓ Be sure to wear proper athletic footwear.
- ✓ Clothes should allow freedom of movement.
- ✓ Be sure to stay well hydrated with water and other fluids through out the day.

✓ Keep a fitness journal to record what exercises you performed each day, how you felt during and after your exercise session, and rate how hard you worked out during your routine (low intensity, medium intensity, or high intensity practice).

What You'll Need To Do These Exercises:

- Exercise step
- Chair

Stair Walking

Position yourself standing in front of an exercise step, feet hip-width apart. Place one foot on the step, and then the other, so that both feet are on the step. Place one foot back on the floor, and then the other foot. Repeat the steps.

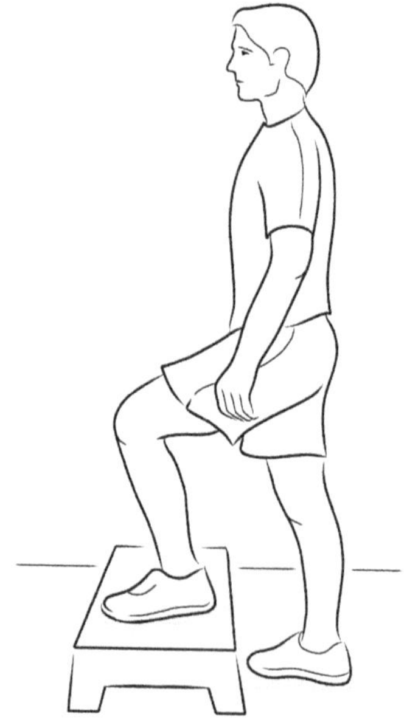

1. STAIR WALKING

Squat

Stand with your feet hip-width apart, toes pointing to eleven o'clock and one o'clock. Place your hands on your knees. Drop you hips as low as possible.

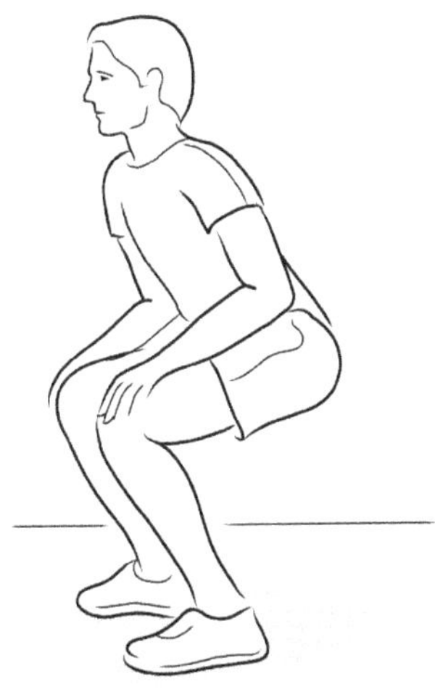

2. SQUAT

Getting Up (From A Chair)

Position yourself on the edge of a chair. Without using your hands, press your feet into the ground and raise yourself up from the chair.

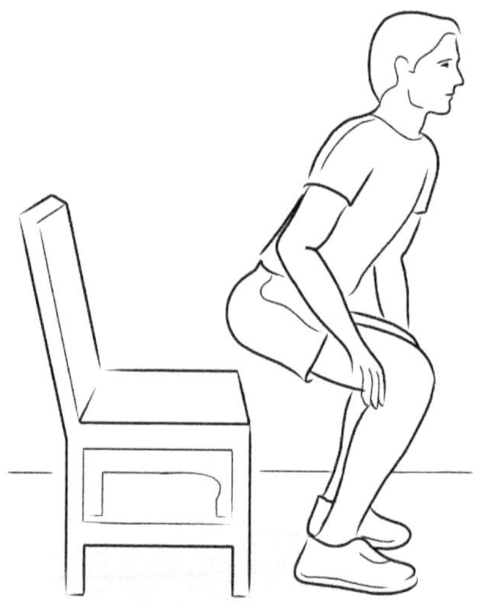

3. GETTING UP

Game Plan Wrap-up

GO, FIGHT, WIN!

Helping people defeat heart disease is more than my profession, it is my passion. It's not about me *making a living*, as much as my patients *living* to the fullest after a diagnosis and treatment plan have been made.

Like a team going over all the plays before the big game, we have covered a lot of significant information in this book. You learned about my own experience as a patient, and how both the patient and the physician must take responsibility when it comes to healing. As a seasoned veteran on both ends of the playing field, I have increased insight and a great commitment to see that all heart patients become winners.

You've learned how the heart works, and what heart disease is. You can recognize threatening symptoms, and know your options for attacking them—so there's no ball fumbling. We reviewed the different modalities used to make a correct diagnosis as well as the terms to explain the pathology. We reviewed the surgical and non-surgical options available.

From there we established that you as a patient are not alone in this fight—that you're one of many players on the bench and on the field. Your caregivers and family play a crucial role in the pre-operative planning, the operation, and the post-operative care. And when it comes to choosing your surgeon and your hospital, you and your family have important choices to make.

Like practicing pre-game drills, we learned how to snap the ball for game day—your surgery. Positive attitude is crucial in preparing for the operation and to ensure an excellent outcome. We want to kick the ball, not the bucket. We laid out the different strategies for dealing with fears and stress, and we formulated a game plan.

We learned in detail what takes place during surgery, as well as what to expect afterwards—both as a patient and as the patient's support team. We discovered that diet and exercise play a crucial role in controlling heart disease, and in maintaining a healthy lifestyle.

Even though I qualify as a successful coach with a great win/loss record, *you* still have as much power to beat heart disease as I do as a physician. I am proud of you for taking this journey with me! We covered lots of ground, from the kick off to the touchdown, and all the locker room training rules in between. I hope that you have gained an understanding of what it takes to carry the ball and get through the game. It is not easy to be a patient, but with the right preparation, good support team, and a positive attitude, you will always win!

ABOUT THE AUTHOR

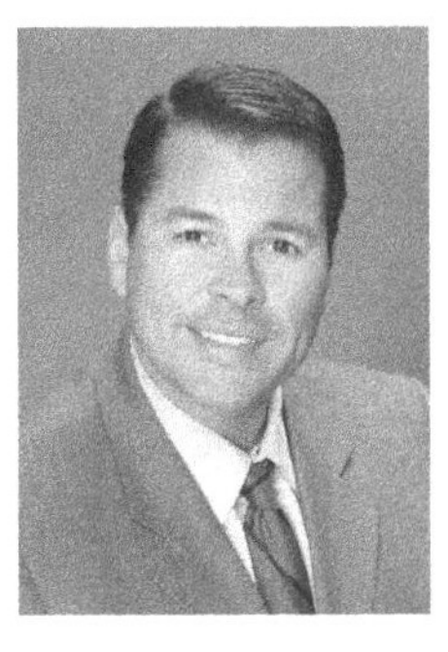

Jacob DeLaRosa, M.D. was raised in Los Angeles, California. The son of a physician, he aspired to be a doctor from an early age. Upon becoming a surgeon, Dr. DeLaRosa quickly learned he didn't fit the traditional mold or expectations of his colleagues. He is a good listener who is fast with a joke and a hug. His patients have embraced his charming and encouraging "coaching" style, and his impressive track record. Dr. DeLaRosa is a board-certified cardiac and thoracic surgeon, as well as a board-certified general surgeon, who specializes in open-heart surgery and endovascular surgery.

He is the Chief of Cardiothoracic and Endovascular Surgery at Portneuf Medical Center. He has received hundreds of awards and honors, and is a professional member of multiple national and international medical societies. Dr. DeLaRosa trained at the University of Minnesota School of Medicine, completed his general surgery residency at the University of California, San Diego Medical Center, and his cardiothoracic surgery training at Emory University in Atlanta, Georgia.

He has been recently featured on the syndicated television show *The Wendy Williams Show* and in *People* magazine. Dr. DeLaRosa is a celebrated speaker in his field, with hundreds of presentations that engage audiences on the topics of cardiac surgery, endovascular surgery, thoracic surgery, self-motivation, and overall heart health throughout the U.S. and internationally. He has authored many peer-reviewed articles in respected medical journals and contributed various chapters for several published medical books.

www.ingramcontent.com/pod-product-compliance
Lightning Source LLC
Chambersburg PA
CBHW070822100426
42813CB00003B/457

9781880759806